Diseases of the Eyes, Ears, Nose & Throat

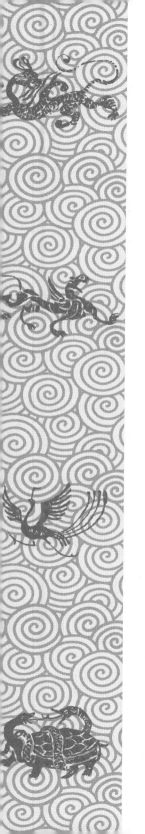

The Treatment of Disease in TCM

VOLUME 2:

Diseases of the Eyes, Ears, Nose & Throat

 by Philippe Sionneau
& Lü Gang

BLUE POPPY PRESS

Published by:

BLUE POPPY PRESS, INC.
1775 LINDEN AVE.
BOULDER, CO 80304

First Edition, June, 1996

ISBN 0-936185-73-2
LC 95-83249

COMP Designation: Original work using a standard translational terminology

Printed at Johnson Printing in Boulder, CO on acid free, recycled, elementally chlorine-free paper

Cover design by Jeff Fuller, Crescent Moon

10 9 8 7 6 5 4 3 2

Author's Foreword

Most TCM textbooks and clinical handbooks describe the diagnosis and treatment of the same major diseases and conditions. These can be either traditional Chinese disease categories, such as lateral costal pain, *shan* qi, and the strangury and turbidity, or they may be modern Western disease diagnoses, such as cholecystitis, chronic appendicitis, Bell's palsy, and endometriosis. However, patients coming to Western acupuncturists or practitioners of Chinese medicine often complain of unpleasant or unusual symptoms which neither modern Western nor contemporary Traditional Chinese Medicine consider diseases in and of themselves. These may include, for instance, dry nose, heavy-headedness, strong smelling armpits, loss of the sense of taste, itchy eyes, coldness in the low back region, tremor of the hands, sweating of the hands, or premature greying of the hair. Thus, these all too commonly encountered complaints do not appear as chapters in our TCM textbooks, and, therefore, we Western practitioners may have trouble finding out about their TCM diagnosis and treatment. Without delving into the Chinese medical literature more deeply, we might even be tempted to say that Chinese medicine does not address many of the complaints of our Western patients.

Being fully aware of this difficulty, when studying in China, I made a special attempt to discover and collect original information on such symptoms or diseases which typically are overlooked in the majority of the literature. My aim was to enlarge our understanding and to widen our knowledge so as to increase our clinical efficacy. This has led me to write the first of this series of practical books for clinical use, classified according to the part of the body where these symptoms appear. These books will cover the main, standard or classical diseases of Chinese medicine as well as a host of other minor diseases and complaints which nonetheless appear often in our real-life patients.

This new approach offers two further advantages besides filling in the gaps in our Western language TCM literature. First, when a patient's major complaint is difficult to diagnose and analyze due to a confused or complicated situation and when a thorough knowledge of the usual methods of diagnosis and of the standard diseases are not sufficient, these nonstandard or little written about symptoms and diseases can help us tackle the problem from a different angle.

For example, if the signs and symptoms of sinusitis or rhinitis in one of our patients do not clearly fall under the usual pattern discrimination of *bi yuan* (deep source nasal congestion), we might find our patient's pattern under dry nose (*bi gan*), nose pain (*bi tong*), itchy nose (*bi yang*), bad odor of the nose (*bi chou*), or acid, sour nose (*bi suan*) if our patient suffers from one of these symptoms. Thus we can approach their case from a slightly different perspective.

The second advantage is that this series of books will offer a new and more exhaustive approach to a number of key symptoms, such as spontaneous perspiration, night sweats, aversion to wind and cold, red cheeks, pale nails, and purple lips. Most current Western language TCM texts only discuss the most basic disease causes and disease mechanisms, patterns and their treatments for these symptoms and conditions, and patients often present with patterns not included in these texts. The causes and mechanisms of these complaints are, in fact, more numerous and varied than most books commonly describe. For example, most books emphasize that night sweats are due to yin vacuity with vacuity heat. But what about heart blood vacuity, spleen vacuity with damp encumbrance, *shao yang* disease, damp heat, and the other causes of night sweats? Or take vexatious heat in the five hearts. It is also typically described as a consequence of yin vacuity and vacuity heat. Whereas, it can just as well be caused by depressive heat in the liver, blood stasis, evils hidden in the yin aspect, heat internally depressed, etc.

Because I am more specialized in internal medicine and Chinese medicinals, I thought it best to ask my friend Lu Gang to compose the acupuncture and moxibustion treatments. When studying in Wuhan, Lu Gang was the person who had the deepest influence on my comprehension of Chinese medicine. He proved to be a competent and efficient guide who helped me reach a more subtle understanding of TCM terminology. Thanks to his outstanding abilities, he obtained a Master of Acupuncture & Moxibustion Degree from the Nanjing College of TCM and has a thorough knowledge of this art. It appeared, therefore, quite logical to ask him to collaborate on this series of books, both in gratitude for the help he has given me in the past and because I was sure his collaboration would enhance the quality of this series.

The terminology in this book is based on Nigel Wiseman's *Glossary of Chinese Medical Terms and Acupuncture Points*, Paradigm Publications, Brookline, MA, 1990 with up-dates and revisions supplied by Nigel Wiseman through Bob Felt of Paradigm Publications. Other divergences from Dr. Wiseman's terminology are noted and discussed in the footnotes.

For further information on the use of processed Chinese medicinals, the reader is referred to my book, *Pao Zhi: An Introduction to the Use of Processed Chinese Medicinals*, also published by Blue Poppy Press. It is my belief that processed medicinals are far more effective than unprocessed medicinals. In TCM, each specific medicinal is identified not only by its species and part or piece but also by its method of processing. Thus, a medicinal consisting of the same part from the same species is a different medicinal if it is processed differently. Obviously, it is extremely important to use the right medicinal in the right situation, and using processed medicinals is, in my opinion, an integral part of using the right medicinal.

All formula dosages are given for a single day's administration unless otherwise stated. In addition, these dosages are for adults. Dosages for children should be adjusted according to their body weight.

Hopefully, this book and the others in this series will help Western practitioners to make progress in the universe of TCM for the benefit of suffering people.

Philippe Sionneau
March 11, 1996
Meras, France

Contents

1
Distention in the Eyes *(Mu Zhang)*

This is a subjective symptom in which the patient feels distention or painful distention in the eyeballs. Sometimes this distention and aching may involve the superciliary arch.

Disease causes, disease mechanisms:

1. Externally contracted wind heat

The foot *tai yang* channel originates from the inner canthus, while the foot *yang ming* channel meets the foot *tai yang* channel at the acupoint, *Jing Ming* (Bl 1). When wind evils are mixed with heat and invade the body, they may go upward along the foot *tai yang* and foot *yang ming* channels and attack the eyes, thus causing blockage there. Hence there is painful distention in the eyeballs which may involve the superciliary arch.

2. Liver depression/qi stagnation

The foot *jue yin* channel connects with the ligation of the eye. Emotional disturbances, such as frustration and anger, may result in liver depression and make the qi stagnant. With time, heat will transform and brew internally. If this heat goes upward along the *jue yin* channel and attacks the eyes, distention and pain in the eyeballs may occur.

3. Dual vacuity of the qi & blood

The heart governs the blood and the spleen is the source of engendering and transformation. If the heart and spleen are damaged by enduring overthinking, the qi and blood will become vacuous. Being vacuous, first, the qi will fail to go upward and warm the eyes, while the blood will fail to nourish the eyes. Secondly, the flow of qi and blood will become slowed-down due to insufficient qi to move the blood. As a result, qi and blood in the region of the eyes will not flow freely and distention in the eyeballs may follow.

Treatment based on pattern discrimination:

I. Externally contracted wind heat

Symptoms: The main complaints include distention in the eyeballs, pain or aching in the superciliary arch when the distention is severe, weak eyelids, and inability to look for a long time. Accompanying symptoms may include fever with aversion to cold, headache, a red tongue with yellow fur, and a floating, rapid pulse.

Therapeutic principles: Course wind and scatter cold

Acupuncture & moxibustion:

Zhan Zhu (Bl 2) A point of the urinary bladder channel; courses wind and opens the network vessels.

Feng Chi (GB 20) A key point for eye problems; it clears the head and eyes.

He Gu (LI 4) Together, these points course wind and clear heat.
Wai Guan (TB 5)

Additions & subtractions: If there is fever, add *Da Zhui* (GV 14). If there is headache, add *Tou Wei* (St 8).

Chinese medicinal formula: *Xiong Ju Shang Qing Wan* (Ligusticum Wallichium & Chrysanthemum Ascend & Clear Pills)

Ingredients: Flos Chrysanthemi Morifolii (*Ju Hua*), 10g, Radix Ligustici Wallichii (*Chuan Xiong*), 10g, Radix Scutellariae Baicalensis (*Huang Qin*), 10g, Radix Angelicae Dahuricae (*Bai Zhi*), 6g, Fructus Gardeniae Jasminoidis (*Zhi Zi*), 6g, Fructus Viticis (*Man Jing Zi*), 10g, Fructus Forsythiae Suspensae (*Lian Qiao*), 10g, Herba Schizonepetae Tenuifoliae (*Jing Jie*), 10g, Radix Platycodi Grandiflori (*Jie Geng*), 6g, Radix Ledebouriellae Divaricatae (*Fang Feng*), 6g, Herba Menthae Haplocalycis (*Bo He*), 3g, Rhizoma Coptidis Chinensis (*Huang Lian*), 3g, Radix Et Rhizoma Notopterygii (*Qiang Huo*), 6g, Radix Et Rhizoma Ligustici Chinensis (*Gao Ben*), 6g

2. Liver depression/qi stagnation

Symptoms: Discomfort and distention in the eyeballs without obvious pain, reddening of the eyes, tearing, or increased eye discharge. Other symptoms may include chest oppression, lateral costal pain, a bitter taste in the mouth, dry throat, a red tongue with thin fur, and a wiry, fine or rapid pulse.

Therapeutic principles: Course the liver and resolve depression, cool the liver and clear heat

Acupuncture & moxibustion:

Feng Chi (GB 20)	Together, these points harmonize the network
Yu Yao (M-HN-6)	vessels and help clear heat in the gallbladder and liver channels.

Xing Jian (Liv 2)	Together, the spring points of the liver and
Xia Xi (GB 43)	gallbladder channels cool the liver and clear heat.

Tai Chong (Liv 3)	Together, the transporting and alarm points of the
Qi Men (Liv 14)	liver channel course the liver and resolve depression.

Additions & subtractions: If there is tearing, add *Tou Lin Qi* (GB 15).

Chinese medicinal formula: *Jia Wei Xiao Yao San* (Added Flavors Rambling Powder)

Ingredients: Cortex Radicis Moutan (*Dan Pi*), 12g, Fructus Gardeniae Jasminoidis (*Zhi Zi*), 10g, Radix Bupleuri (*Chai Hu*), 6g, Radix Albus Paeoniae Lactiflorae (*Bai Shao*), 10g, Rhizoma Atractylodis Macrocephalae (*Bai Zhu*), 10g, Sclerotium Poriae Cocos (*Fu Ling*), 6g, mix-fried Radix Glycyrrhizae (*Zhi Gan Cao*), 3g

3. Dual vacuity of the qi & blood

Symptoms: Distention in the eyeballs which is worsened by overwork or during menstruation in women, a sallow yellow facial complexion, pale lips and nails, heart palpitations, insomnia, shortness of breath, spontaneous perspiration, a pale tongue, and a fine, weak pulse

Therapeutic principles: Boost the qi and nourish the blood

Acupuncture & moxibustion:

Feng Chi (GB 20)   Together, these points fortify the spleen to promote
Pi Shu (Bl 20)   the engendering and transformation of qi and blood
Gan Shu (Bl 18)   and supplement liver blood to nourish the eyes.

Chinese medicinal formula: *Chai Hu Shen Zhu Tang* (Bupleurum, Ginseng & Actractylodes Decoction)

Ingredients: Radix Bupleuri (*Chai Hu*), 6g, Radix Panacis Ginseng (*Ren Shen*), 6g, Rhizoma Atractylodis Macrocephalae (*Bai Zhu*), 12g, prepared Radix Rehmanniae (*Shu Di*), 12g, Radix Albus Paeoniae Lactiflorae (*Bai Shao*), 10g, Radix Angelicae Sinensis (*Dang Gui*), 10g, Pericarpium Citri Reticulatae Viride (*Qing Pi*), 6g, Radix Ligustici Wallichii (*Chuan Xiong*), 6g, mix-fried Radix Glycyrrhizae (*Zhi Gan Cao*), 3g

2
Itchy Eyes *(Mu Yang)*

This is a symptom of itching on the margins of the eyelids and inner canthi. When severe, this itching may involve the conjunctiva, becoming unbearable. Nevertheless, the vision is not affected. This category does not cover itching as a secondary or concomitant symptom in other patterns.

Disease causes, disease mechanisms:

Wind is always the cause of itching. As it is said in Chinese medicine, "No wind, no itching."

I. Invasion of wind evils

If externally contracted wind enters the canthi and travels back and forth in between the interstices, this may cause itching.

2. Externally contracted wind heat

On the cusp of spring and summer, yang is becoming predominant and the liver (spring) is giving way to the heart (summer). If external wind heat invades the body during this time, it is likely to attack the liver channel and the exterior/interior correlated gallbladder channel. The liver channel connects with the eyes. When wind heat invasion attacks upward along this channel, itching in the eyes may follow.

3. Externally contracted wind cold

The disease causes and disease mechanisms are essentially the same for wind cold as for wind heat since, in both cases, it is the wind that is specifically causing the itching.

4. Fire exuberance

Fire can be the result of externally contracted evils, emotional disturbances, dietary irregularity, etc. Fire's nature is to flame upward. Wind by its nature tends to attack the upper part of the body. If fire already exists, an externally contracted wind may trigger its upward attack. If the eyes are affected, itching may occur there.

5. Damp heat brewing internally

Damp heat may brew internally if the spleen and stomach are damaged due to dietary irregularity. In such an abnormal condition, an externally contracted wind may lead this damp heat upward along the channels. When the evils affect the eyes, itching may occur as a result.

6. Liver blood vacuity

Liver blood vacuity may arise as a result of general blood vacuity, aging, and extended use of the eyes which consumes the blood, as in reading. Blood vacuity may render the liver blood vacuous and engender wind. On the one hand, the eyes will be undernourished due to liver blood vacuity, and, on the other, wind due to blood vacuity may attack the eyes along the liver channel. Thus itching may occur in the eyes.

Treatment based on pattern discrimination:

I. Invasion of wind evils

Symptoms: Itching in the canthi with normal vision. No other symptoms may be observed.

Therapeutic principles: Dispel wind and stop itching

Acupuncture & moxibustion:

Feng Chi (GB 20)   A key point to dispel wind so as to stop itching

Zan Zhu (Bl 2)   Together, these points course wind in the foot *tai*
Tou Wei (St 8)   *yang* and foot *yang ming* channels.

Tai Yang (M-HN-9)   Helps the above three points course wind to stop
                              itching

Note: The needles should be pointed towards the area of the eyes. If the itching is severe, prick *Tai Yang* and *Tou Wei* to induce bleeding.

Chinese medicinal formula: *Qu Feng San* (Dispel Wind Powder)

Ingredients: Herba Menthae Haplocalycis (*Bo He*), 3g, Radix Ledebouriellae Divaricatae (*Fang Feng*), 10g, Radix Et Rhizoma Notopterygii (*Qiang Huo*), 10g, Herba Schizonepetae Tenuifoliae (*Jing Jie*), 10g, Radix Ligustici Wallichii (*Chuan Xiong*), 10g, Radix Aconiti Carmichaeli (*Chuan Wu Tou*), 3g

2. Externally contracted wind heat

Symptoms: Unbearable itching as if there were insects in the eyes, a local sensation of burning heat, slight photophobia and tearing, scant eye discharge with spinbarkeit and red granules inside the eyelids. This type of itching is mainly seen in young people in the spring and can be exacerbated by wind, sun, and exposure to fire and smoke. Other symptoms are thin, white tongue fur and a floating, rapid pulse.

Therapeutic principles: Course wind and clear heat, quicken the blood and dispel stasis

Acupuncture & moxibustion:

Feng Chi (GB 20)   Together, these points course wind and clear heat.
Tai Yang (M-HN-9)

7

Si Bai (St 2) *He Gu* (LI 4)	Together, these points drain heat by draining the *yang ming* channel which is rich qi and blood.
Tong Zi Liao (GB 1) *Di Wu Hui* (GB 42)	Together, these points clear heat in the *shao yang* channel by matching points above and below.
Shao Shang (Lu 11)	When pricked to induce bleeding, quickens the blood and dispels stasis. In addition, it helps the other points to course wind heat.

Chinese medicinal formula: Modified *Si Wu Tang* (Four Materials Decoction)

Ingredients: Fructus Arctii Lappae (*Niu Bang Zi*), 10g, Herba Schizonepetae Tenuifoliae (*Jing Jie*), 10g, Radix Ledebouriellae Divaricatae (*Fang Feng*), 10g, Fructus Forsythiae Suspensae (*Lian Qiao*), 10g, Herba Menthae Haplocalycis (*Bo He*), 3g, Radix Ligustici Wallichii (*Chuan Xiong*), 10g, uncooked Radix Rehmanniae (*Sheng Di*), 6g, Radix Sophorae Flavescentis (*Ku Shen*), 6g, Radix Trichosanthis Kirlowii (*Tian Hua Fen*), 6g, Radix Rubrus Paeoniae Lactiflorae (*Chi Shao*), 10g, Radix Angelicae Sinensis (*Dang Gui*), 6g

3. Externally contracted wind cold

Symptoms: Itchy eyes exacerbated by cold wind, tearing and thin eye discharge. No eye screen or organic abnormality can be observed. The vision is normal. Other possible symptoms include aching around the supraorbital bone, aversion to cold, nasal congestion, thin, white tongue fur, and a floating, wiry pulse.

Therapeutic principles: Expel wind, scatter cold, and stop itching

Acupuncture & moxibustion:

See the prescription for externally contracted wind heat above.

Additions & subtractions: If there is aching around the supraorbital bone, add *Yu Yao* (M-HN-6). If there is marked aversion to cold, add *Wai Guan* (TB 5).

Chinese medicinal formula: Modified *Ren Shen Qiang Huo Tang* (Ginseng & Notopterygium Decoction)

Ingredients: Radix Panacis Ginseng (*Ren Shen*), 3g, Sclerotium Poriae Cocos (*Fu Ling*), 6g, Radix Et Rhizoma Notopterygii (*Qiang Huo*), 10g, Radix Angelicae Pubescentis (*Du Huo*), 10g, Radix Ligustici Wallichii (*Chai Hu*), 10g, Radix Bupleuri (*Chai Hu*), 3g, Radix Platycodi Grandiflori (*Jie Geng*), 3g, Radix Peucedani (*Qian Hu*), 6g, Bombyx Batryticatus (*Jiang Can*), 12g, Radix Aconiti Carmichaeli (*Chuan Wu Tou*), 3g

4. Fire exuberance

Symptoms: Severe itching with a sensation of burning heat, redness of the whites of the eyes, hot tears, thick eye discharge, dryness and a bitter taste in the mouth, dark-colored urine, dry stools, a red tongue with yellow fur, and a rapid pulse

Therapeutic principles: Downbear fire, discharge heat, and stop itching

Acupuncture & moxibustion:

Tong Zi Liao (GB 1)	Together, these points clear heat when pricked to
Zan Zhu (Bl 2)	induce bleeding.
Feng Chi (GB 20)	A point of the gallbladder channel which drains heat in the channel
Xing Jian (Liv 2)	The spring point of the liver channel; downbears and drains heat in its channel
He Gu (LI 4)	The source point of the hand *yang ming* channel; clears heat in the head and the eyes

Additions & subtractions: If there are hot tears, add *Cheng Qi* (St 1).

Chinese medicinal formula: *Liang Ge San* (Cool the Diaphragm Powder)

Ingredients: Fructus Forsythiae Suspensae (*Lian Qiao*), 12g, Radix Et Rhizoma Rhei (*Da Huang*), 6g, Mirabilitum (*Mang Xiao*), 6g, Fructus Gardeniae Jasminoidis (*Zhi Zi*), 6g, Radix Scutellariae Baicalensis (*Huang Qin*), 10g, Herba Menthae Haplocalycis (*Bo He*), 3g, Folium Bambusae (*Zhu Ye*), 6g, Radix Glycyrrhizae (*Gan Cao*), 3g

5. Damp heat brewing internally

Symptoms: Unbearably itchy eyes, sticky tears and eye discharge, heavy eyelids, yellow turbidity in the whites of the eyes, slimy, yellow tongue fur, and a soggy pulse

Therapeutic principles: Dispel wind and clear heat, eliminate dampness and stop itching

Acupuncture & moxibustion:

Cheng Qi (St 1)   Together, these points dispel wind and clear heat,
Qu Chi (LI 11)   open the network vessels in the eyes and stop itching.
Tai Yang (M-HN-9)

Zu San Li (St 36)   Fortifies spleen and transforms dampness

Feng Long (St 40)   Eliminates dampness

Chinese medicinal formula: Modified *Chu Shi Tang* (Eliminate Dampness Decoction)

Ingredients: Fructus Forsythiae Suspensae (*Lian Qiao*), 10g, Semen Plantaginis (*Che Qian Zi*), 10g, Fructus Citri Aurantii (*Zhi Ke*), 6g, Radix Scutellariae Baicalensis (*Huang Qin*), 10g, Rhizoma Coptidis

Chinensis (*Huang Lian*), 6g, Caulis Akebiae (*Mu Tong*), 5g, Pericarpium Citri Reticulatae (*Chen Pi*), 10g, Sclerotium Poriae Cocos (*Fu Ling*), 10g, Radix Ledebouriellae Divaricatae (*Fang Feng*), 10g, Zaocys Dhumnades (*Wu Xiao She*), 5g, Periostracum Cicadae (*Chan Tui*), 10g, Radix Ligustici Wallichii (*Chuan Xiong*), 10g, Radix Et Rhizoma Notopterygii (*Qiang Huo*), 10g

6. Liver blood vacuity

Symptoms: Minor itching relieved by kneading the eyes and reoccurring on release, dry, rough eyes, a lusterless facial complexion, a pale tongue, and a wiry, fine pulse

Therapeutic principles: Nourish and quicken the blood, extinguish wind and stop itching

Acupuncture & moxibustion:

Gan Shu (Bl 18)   Together, these points supplement the liver and
Xue Hai (Sp 10)   nourish the blood to extinguish wind.

Bai Hui (GV 20)   Leads the qi and blood upward to nourish the eyes

Feng Chi (GB 20)   Together, these points help lead the qi and blood
Tong Zi Liao (GB 1)   upward to nourish the eyes and extinguish wind.

Chinese medicinal formula: Modified *Si Wu Tang* (Four Materials Decoction)

Ingredients: Prepared Radix Rehmanniae (*Shu Di*), 15g, Radix Albus Paeoniae Lactiflorae (*Bai Shao*), 12g, Radix Angelicae Sinensis (*Dang Gui*), 10g, Radix Ligustici Wallichii (*Chuan Xiong*), 10g, Radix Ledebouriellae Divaricatae (*Fang Feng*), 10g, Buthus Martensi (*Quan Xie*), 3g, Radix Aconiti Carmichaeli (*Chuan Wu Tou*), 5g

3
Clouded Vision *(Mu Hun)*

This refers to dimness of the vision.

Disease causes, disease mechanisms:

I. Wind phlegm harassing above

Dampness may be due to spleen vacuity in turn due to dietary irregularity and an exuberant liver which overwhelms the spleen. If accumulated dampness endures, it will engender heat with time. This heat will then steam this dampness into phlegm. The exuberant liver will give rise to hyperactivity of upbearing and effusing and thus induce wind. If wind and phlegm go upward to harass the clear portals, the vision may be clouded.

2. Liver depression/qi stagnation

Depression and anger may damage the liver and lead to failure of the liver's orderly reaching. The liver channel connects with the ligation of the eyes. Thus, if liver qi counterflows upward along the channel to harass the eyes, clouded vision may occur.

3. Blood vacuity of the liver & heart

Blood vacuity of the liver and heart may result from great loss of the blood, spleen/stomach vacuity, overthinking, extended reading, etc. The liver stores, while the heart governs the blood. If there is liver blood vacuity, the eyes will be undernourished, since "The liver opens to the eyes" and "The eyes are able to see only when the liver receives sufficient blood." If there is heart blood vacuity, the heart cannot circulate the blood normally, and thus the eyes may be deprived of sufficient nourishment. This is based on the saying, "The heart governs the blood." In such cases, clouded vision may occur.

4. Spleen qi vacuity

Spleen qi vacuity can result from overthinking, dietary irregularity, severe disease, etc. Damaged by the above-mentioned factors, the spleen's function of movement and transformation will become abnormal. First, the spleen will fail to distribute the essence of the viscera and bowels to the eyes. Secondly, less blood and qi will be engendered and transformed. And third, the spleen qi may fail to upbear clear yang qi to warm the eyes. As a result, the vision may become clouded.

5. Yin vacuity of the liver & kidneys

Yin vacuity of the liver and kidneys may result from sexual taxation, multiple births, aging, or severe or chronic diseases. In this case, yin vacuity of the liver and kidneys implies liver blood and kidney essence. Therefore, the eyes will not be properly nourished and clouded vision may occur since the liver and kidneys are responsible for the cornea and the pupil respectively.

6. Debility of the life-gate fire

Debility of the life-gate fire may result from aging, taxation, chronic disease, and original qi consumption. The debilitation may result in 1) poor engendering and transformation of the qi and blood, since the normal function of the spleen and stomach depends on the warming by the life-gate fire, and 2) blockage of the network vessels in the eyes, since normal blood flow also depends on the warming and freeing function of the life-gate fire. In other words, if the life-gate fire becomes debilitated, the eyes will be deprived of sufficient nourishment and the vessels will be blocked due to slow flow of water or blood. As a result, clouded vision may occur.

Treatment based on pattern discrimination:

I. Wind phlegm harassing the upper

Symptoms: Clouded and flowery, *i.e.*, blurred, vision, twitching of the eyelids, dizziness, chest oppression, reduced food intake, profuse sleeping, nausea and vomiting with profuse phlegm, slimy, white tongue fur, and a wiry, slippery pulse

Therapeutic principles: Course wind, transform phlegm, and brighten the eyes

Acupuncture & moxibustion:

Cheng Qi (St 1)	A meeting point of the foot *yang ming*, yang motility vessel, and the conception vessel
Jing Ming (Bl 1)	A meeting point of the *tai yang*, foot *yang ming* channel, yin and yang motility vessels. Together, these points course wind and open the network vessels in the eyes.

He Gu (LI 4) *Feng Chi* (GB 20)	Together, these points course wind, clear the head, and brighten the eyes.

Zu San Li (St 36) *Feng Long* (St 40)	Together, these points fortify the spleen to move the qi and transform phlegm.

Chinese medicinal formula: *Ban Xia Tian Ma Bai Zhu Tang* (Pinellia, Gastrodia & Atractylodes Decoction)

Ingredients: Rhizoma Pinelliae Ternatae (*Ban Xia*), 10g, Rhizoma Atractylodis Macrocephalae (*Bai Zhu*), 15g, Rhizoma Gastrodiae Elatae (*Tian Ma*),10g, Sclerotium Poriae Cocos (*Fu Ling*), 10g, Pericarpium Citri Reticulatae (*Chen Pi*), 10g, mix-fried Radix Glycyrrhizae (*Zhi Gan Cao*), 3g

2. Liver depression/qi stagnation

Symptoms: Clouded vision, distention in the eyes, dizziness, a bitter taste in the mouth, emotional depression, pain in the lateral costal regions, a red tongue with white fur, and a wiry, rapid pulse

Therapeutic principles: Course the liver, resolve depression, and brighten the eyes

Acupuncture & moxibustion:

Qiu Hou (M-HN-8)	An empirical point for vision problems
Tong Zi Liao (GB 1)	A meeting point of the small intestine, triple burner, and gallbladder channels
Feng Chi (GB 20)	A meeting point of the gallbladder and yang linking vessel
	Together, these points free the flow of qi and blood in the eyes.
Tai Chong (Liv 3)	The source point of the liver
Qi Men (Liv 14)	The alarm point of the liver
	Together, these points course the liver, resolve depression, and brighten the eyes.

Chinese medicinal formula: *Xiao Yao San Yan Fang* (Rambling Powder Experiential Formula)

Ingredients: Radix Angelicae Sinensis (*Dang Gui*), 10g, Rhizoma Atractylodis Macrocephalae (*Bai Zhu*), 12g, Radix Albus Paeoniae Lactiflorae (*Bai Shao*), 10g, Cortex Radicis Moutan (*Dan Pi*), 6g, Sclerotium Poriae Cocos (*Fu Ling*), 6g, Fructus Gardeniae Jasminoidis (*Zhi Zi*), 6g, Flos Chrysanthemi Morifolii (*Ju Hua*), 10g, Fructus Lycii Chinensis (*Gou Qi Zi*), 12g, Rhizoma Acori Graminei (*Shi Chang Pu*), 6g, Radix Glycyrrhizae (*Gan Cao*), 3g

3. Blood vacuity of the heart & liver

Symptoms: Indistinct vision with dry, rough eyes which are exacerbated by overwork. Other symptoms may include a lusterless facial complexion, heart palpitations, insomnia, a pale tongue and lips, and a fine, forceless pulse.

Therapeutic principles: Supplement the blood, nourish the liver, and brighten the eyes

Acupuncture & moxibustion:

Feng Chi (GB 20)   Together, these points free the flow of qi and
Cheng Qi (St 1)   blood in the eyes.
Qiu Hou (M-HN-8)

Xin Shu (Bl 15)   Together, these points supplement heart/liver
Gan Shu (Bl 18)   blood to nourish the eyes.
Pi Shu (Bl 20)

Chinese medicinal formula: *Si Wu Tang* (Four Materials Decoction) plus Modified *Bu Xin Dan* (Supplement the Heart Elixir)

Ingredients: Prepared Radix Rehmanniae (*Shi Di*), 12g, Radix Albus Paeoniae Lactiflorae (*Bai Shao*), 10g, Radix Ligustici Wallichii (*Chuan Xiong*), 6g, Radix Angelicae Sinensis (*Dang Gui*), 12g, Tuber Ophiopogonis Japonici (*Mai Dong*), 12g, Tuber Asparagi Cochinensis (*Tian Dong*), 12g, Radix Polygalae Tenuifoliae (*Yuan Zhi*), 10g, Rhizoma Acori Graminei (*Shi Chang Pu*), 6g, Rhizoma Atractylodis Macrocephalae (*Bai Zhu*), 10g, Sclerotium Pararadicis Poriae Cocos (*Fu Shen*), 10g

4. Spleen qi vacuity

Symptoms: Indistinct vision, weak eyelids, fatigue of the eyes when used for extended periods, a sallow yellow facial complexion, fatigue, lack of strength, scant food intake, loose stools, a slightly red tongue with thin, white fur, and a vacuous, weak pulse

Therapeutic principles: Fortify the spleen, supplement the qi, and brighten the eyes

Acupuncture & moxibustion:

Cheng Qi (St 1)	Together, these points free the flow of qi and
Qiu Hou (M-HN-8)	blood in the eyes.
Bai Hui (GV 20)	With moxibustion, upbears the qi
He Gu (LI 4)	Together, these points supplement the qi.
Zu San Li (St 36)	

Additions & subtractions: Add *Qi Hai* (CV 6) if there is severe qi vacuity. In that case, moxibustion is suggested.

Chinese medicinal formula: *Bu Zhong Yi Qi Tang* (Supplement the Center & Boost the Qi Decoction)

Ingredients: Radix Astragali Membranacei (*Huang Qi*), 12g, Rhizoma Atractylodis Macrocephalae (*Bai Zhu*), 15g, Radix Panacis Ginseng (*Ren Shen*), 5g, Radix Angelicae Sinensis (*Dang Gui*), 6g, Pericarpium Citri Reticulatae (*Chen Pi*), 6g, Radix Bupleuri (*Chai Hu*), 3g, Rhizoma Cimicifugae (*Sheng Ma*), 3g, mix-fried Radix Glycyrrhizae (*Zhi Gan Cao*), 6g

5. Yin vacuity of the liver & kidneys

Symptoms: Indistinct vision, dry, rough eyes, dizziness, tinnitus, low back and knee pain and weakness, seminal emission, night sweats, a dry, painful throat, a red tongue, and a fine, rapid pulse

Therapeutic principles: Nourish and supplement the liver and kidneys, brighten the eyes

Acupuncture & moxibustion:

Feng Chi (GB 20) *Qiu Hou* (M-HN-8)	Together, these points brighten the eyes.
Gan Shu (Bl 18) *Shen Shu* (Bl 23) *Tai Xi* (Ki 3)	Together, these points enrich and supplement liver/kidney yin.
Guang Ming (GB 37)	The network point of the gallbladder; regulates the liver and brightens the eyes

Chinese medicinal formula: Modified *Zuo Gui Wan* (Restore the Left [Kidney] Pills)

Ingredients: Prepared Radix Rehmanniae (*Shu Di*), 10g, Radix Dioscoreae Oppositae (*Shan Yao*), 10g, Fructus Lycii Chinensis (*Gou Qi Zi*), 15g, Fructus Corni Officinalis (*Shan Zhu Yu*), 10g, Radix Achyranthis Bidentatae (*Huai Niu Xi*), 10g, Semen Cuscutae Chinesis (*Tu Si Zi*), 12g, Gelatinum Cornu Cervi (*Lu Jiao Jiao*), 5g, Gelatinum Plastri Testudinis (*Gui Ban Jiao*), 5g, Fructus Ligustri Lucidi (*Nu Zhen Zi*), 12g

6. Debility of the life-gate fire

Symptoms: Dimming of the vision, a drained white facial complexion, cold body and chilled limbs, impotence, premature ejaculation, spontaneous perspiration, frequent urination at night, and a deep, fine, forceless pulse

Therapeutic principles: Warm and supplement the life-gate fire and brighten the eyes

Acupuncture & moxibustion:

Feng Chi (GB 20)   Together, these points free the flow of qi and
Cheng Qi (St 1)   blood in the eyes.

Bai Hui (GV 20)   Together, these points warm and supplement life-
Qi Hai Shu (Bl 24)   gate fire.
Guan Yuan Shu (Bl 26)
Ming Men (GV 4)

Note: Moxibustion should be applied on the last four points after acupuncture.

Chinese medicinal formula: Modified *You Gui Wan* (Restore the Right [Kidney] Pills)

Ingredients: Prepared Radix Rehmanniae (*Shu Di*), 10g, Radix Dioscoreae Oppositae (*Shan Yao*), 10g, Fructus Corni Officinalis (*Shan Zhu Yu*), 10g, Fructus Lycii Chinensis (*Gou Qi Zi*), 12g, Semen Cuscutae Chinesis (*Tu Si Zi*), 12g, Semen Astragali Complanati (*Sha Yuan Zi*), 12g, Fructus Rubi Chingii (*Fu Pen Zi*), 12g, Radix Angelicae Sinensis (*Dang Gui*), 6g, Gelatinum Cornu Cervi (*Lu Jiao Jiao*), 5g, Cortex Cinnamomi Cassiae (*Rou Gui*), 3g

Remarks: Although acupuncture is effective for clouded vision, its effect will not be remarkable before at least 3 months of treatment.

4
Rough Eyes *(Mu Se)*

Rough eyes refers to a feeling of dryness and roughness due to lack of fluids lubricating the eyes.

Disease causes, disease mechanisms:

I. Yin debility & blood vacuity

Yin debility and blood vacuity may arise from: 1) Enduring reading. This is based on the saying, "Extended looking damages the blood." 2) Addiction to alcoholic beverages and sexual taxation which can render yin essence vacuous. 3) Enduring crying due to grief. This exhausts the humors. And 4) anxiety and overthinking may damage the spleen and render the source of engendering and transforming insufficient. If there is yin debility and blood vacuity, the eyes will not be properly lubricated with fluids and are not sufficiently nourished by the blood. Thus rough eyes may occur.

2. Dry heat damaging liquids

Externally contracted dry heat mainly affects the lungs. Lung metal, when exuberant, may overwhelm liver wood. Dryness is a yang evil that can easily damage liquids. The liver channel connects with the ligation of the eyes, and the liver opens into the portal of the eyes. If dryness is contracted, this may damage liquids and involve liver yin. Hence the eyes will not be lubricated or nourished properly. Therefore, rough eyes may occur.

Treatment based on pattern discrimination:

I. Yin debility & blood vacuity

Symptoms: Dryness and scant liquids in the eyes, discomfort of the eyes, a rough sensation in the eyes, easy fatigue of the eyes when looking, a sallow yellow facial complexion, pale nails, insomnia, profuse dreaming, dizziness, tinnitus, a dry tongue and throat, possible vexatious heat in the five hearts, possible low back ache and seminal emission, a pale or red tongue with scant fur, and a fine, rapid pulse

Therapeutic principles: Nourish the kidneys and liver, supplement the blood and moisten dryness

Acupuncture & moxibustion:

Jing Ming (Bl 1) Together, these points free the flow of fluids and
Zan Zhu (Bl 2) blood in the eyes.

Gan Shu (Bl 18) Together, these points supplement the liver and
Pi Shu (Bl 20) spleen to foster yin and nourish the blood.

San Yin Jiao (Sp 6) A meeting point of the three yin channels
Tai Xi (Ki 3) The source point of the kidney channel
Together, these points strongly nourish yin liquids to moisten the eyes.

Chinese medicinal formula: *Si Wu Wu Zi Wan* (Four Materials Schizandra Pills)

Ingredients: Radix Angelicae Sinensis (*Dang Gui*), 10g, prepared Radix Rehmanniae (*Shu Di*), 12g, Radix Albus Paeoniae Lactiflorae (*Bai Shao*), 10g, Radix Ligustici Wallichii (*Chuan Xiong*), 6g, Semen Plantaginis (*Che Qian Zi*), 10g, Fructus Rubi Chingii (*Fu Pen Zi*), 10g, Fructus Lycii Chinensis (*Gou Qi Zi*), 12g, Semen Cuscutae Chinesis (*Tu Si Zi*),

12g, Fructus Kochiae Scopariae (*Di Fu Zi*), 6g

2. Dry heat damaging liquids

Symptoms: Dry, hot, itchy eyes, a rough sensation in the eyes, a dry cough with scanty phlegm, a dry mouth and throat, thirst with desire for liquids, a red tongue with scanty liquids, and a rapid pulse

Therapeutic principles: Clear heat and moisten dryness

Acupuncture & moxibustion:

Si Bai (St 2)   Together, these points clear heat in the eyes.
Tong Zi Liao (GB 1)

Tai Yuan (Lu 9)   The source point of the lungs
Chi Ze (Lu 5)   The sea point of the lungs
                        Together, these points clear lung heat when needled with draining method.

Fu Liu (Ki 7)   Together, these points engender liquids to moisten
San Yin Jiao (Sp 6)   dryness when needled with supplementing method.

Chinese medicinal formula: *Qing Zao Jiu Fei Tang* (Clear Dryness & Rescue the Lungs Decoction)

Ingredients: Folium Mori Albi (*Sang Ye*), 12g, Gypsum Fibrosum (*Shi Gao*), 20g, Radix Panacis Ginseng (*Ren Shen*), 6g, black Semen Sesami Indici (*Hei Zhi Ma*), 10g, Gelatinum Corii Asini (*E Jiao*), 5g, Tuber Ophiopogonis Japonici (*Mai Dong*), 10g, Semen Pruni Armeniacae (*Xing Ren*), 10g, Folium Eriobotryae Japonicae (*Pi Pa Ye*), 10g, Radix Glycyrrhizae (*Gan Cao*), 6g

5
Swollen Eyelids *(Mu Bao Zhong Zhang)*

This refers to swelling with either red or normal colored skin of the upper or both eyelids. This is accompanied by a feeling of distention and discomfort.

Disease causes, disease mechanisms:

The eyelids pertain to the spleen and thus spleen abnormality is very often at fault in this condition. In general, swollen eyelids are categorized as either a repletion or vacuity pattern. The former is mainly due to the heat of damp heat rising upward, while the latter is mainly from yang and qi vacuity failing to move and transform liquids properly.

I. Accumulated heat in the lungs & spleen

Accumulated heat in the lungs and spleen mainly develops from externally contracted wind heat or toxic evils or from dietary irregularity, such as addiction to alcohol, or hot, spicy, and greasy, fatty foods. If this accumulated heat goes upward, as is its wont, and remains in the eyelids, swelling of the eyelids may occur.

2. Attack from liver fire & damp heat

Liver fire mainly arises from emotional disturbances. Based on the saying, "The liver likes orderly reaching," emotional depression and frustration may result in liver depression and stagnant qi. With time, this may transform into fire. Because "The liver's nature is to upbear and effuse," if emotional disturbance such as anger causes hyperactivity of upbearing and effusing, this may then result in the engendering of fire. In addition, if the liver is exuberant, it will overwhelm the spleen, rendering the spleen vacuous. When it becomes vacuous, the spleen may fail in its function of movement and transformation and this may ultimately cause accumulation of dampness. In this case, liver fire may combine with dampness and then go upward to attack the eyes. Thus swollen eyelids may occur.

3. Qi vacuity of the spleen & lungs

Spleen qi vacuity may occur when there is dietary irregularity, overthinking, taxation, enduring disease, and constitutional insufficiency, while lung qi vacuity may arise from enduring grief and chronic cough. Water dampness will accumulate internally if the spleen's function of movement and transformation is impaired due to spleen qi vacuity, and water dampness will not be distributed properly if there is blockage of the water passageways due to lung qi vacuity. If this water dampness collects in the eyelids, there will be swelling there.

4. Yang vacuity of the spleen & kidneys

Yang vacuity of the spleen and kidneys can be the result of constitutional vacuity, severe or chronic disease, or taxation. With yang vacuity, water dampness is not warmed and transformed properly and thus may accumulate internally. The eyelids pertain to the spleen. If accumulated dampness floods in the upper body, the eyelids may, therefore, swell.

5. Dual vacuity of the heart & spleen

Overthinking is often to blame for vacuity of the heart and spleen. Dampness will tend to accumulate internally when the spleen becomes vacuous and fails in its function of movement and transformation. Further, this dampness will not be warmed and transformed properly if heart yang fails to support spleen yang to do so. In other words, when there is a yang vacuity of the heart and spleen, dampness accumulation will follow. And, if dampness collects in the eyelids, there will be swelling there.

Treatment based on pattern discrimination:

I. Accumulated heat in the lungs & spleen

Symptoms: At the early stage, the symptoms are red eyes, hot tears at times, and photophobia followed by swollen eyelids which look like a red peach. Pain is exacerbated on pressure and sometimes refers to the forehead. In some cases, fever with aversion to cold may be seen. Other symptoms are a red tongue and a rapid pulse.

Therapeutic principles: Clear heat, dissipate wind, and resolve toxins

Acupuncture & moxibustion:

Feng Chi (GB 20)   Together, these points dissipate wind and clear
He Gu (LI 4)   the eyes.

Shang Xing (GV 23) Together, these points clear the eyes, resolve
Tai Yang (M-HN-9)   toxins, and disperse swelling when pricked to
Yu Yao (M-HN-6)   induce bleeding.

Additions & subtractions: If there is a high fever, add *Da Zhui* (GV 14).

Chinese medicinal formula: *San Re Xiao Du Yin* (Dissipate Heat & Disperse Toxins Drink)

Ingredients: Fructus Arctii Lappae (*Niu Bang Zi*), 12g, Radix Et Rhizoma Notopterygii (*Qiang Huo*),10g, Rhizoma Coptidis Chinensis (*Chuan Lian*), 6g, Radix Scutellariae Baicalensis (*Huang Qin*), 10g, Herba Menthae Haplocalycis (*Bo He*), 3g, Fructus Forsythiae Suspensae (*Lian Qiao*), 12g

2. Attack from liver fire & damp heat

Symptoms: Severe swelling of the eyelids, inability to open the eyes, redness of the eyelids, a bitter taste in the mouth, distention of the eyes, headache, a red tongue with slimy fur, and a wiry, rapid pulse

Therapeutic principles: Drain the liver, clear heat, and disinhibit dampness

Acupuncture & moxibustion:

Feng Chi (GB 20)	First, drains heat in the gallbladder and, secondly, with *He Gu* (LI 4) clears heat in the head and eyes
Tong Zi Liao (GB 1) *Zan Zhu* (Bl 2)	Together, these points clear heat, transform stasis, and disperse swelling when pricked to induce bleeding.
Shao Shang (Lu 11)	One of the 12 well points; drains heat and cools blood when pricked to induce bleeding
Xing Jian (Liv 2) *Yin Ling Quan* (Sp 9)	The spring point of the liver The sea point of the spleen Together, these points drain the liver, clear heat, and disinhibit dampness.

Chinese medicinal formula: Modified *Long Dan Xie Gan Tang* (Gentiana Drain the Liver Decoction)

Ingredients: Radix Gentianae Scabrae (*Long Dan Cao*), 6g, Caulis Akebiae (*Mu Tong*), 5g, Rhizoma Alismatis (*Ze Xie*), 10g, Semen Plantaginis (*Che Qian Zi*), 10g, uncooked Radix Rehmanniae (*Sheng Di*), 10g, Radix Angelicae Sinensis (*Dang Gui*), 6g, Fructus Gardeniae Jasminoidis (*Zhi Zi*), 6g, Radix Scutellariae Baicalensis (*Huang Qin*), 6g, Radix Bupleuri (*Chai Hu*), 3g, Flos Lonicerae Japonicae (*Jin Yin Hua*), 10g, Fructus Forsythiae Suspensae (*Lian Qiao*), 10g, Radix Glycyrrhizae (*Gan Cao*), 3g

3. Qi vacuity of the spleen & lungs

Symptoms: Swelling in the eyelids, especially in the upper eyelid, which can be relieved somewhat by pressure but soon returns on releasing the pressure, normal skin color, no pain or redness in the eyes, in some cases, itchy eyes, a fat tongue with thin, white fur, and a weak pulse

Therapeutic principles: Supplement the center and boost the qi, fortify the spleen and percolate dampness

Acupuncture & moxibustion:

Wai Guan (TB 5)	The network point of the triple burner; frees and regulates the water passageways
He Gu (LI 4)	The source point of the large intestine
	Together, these points move the qi to disinhibit water.
Zu San Li (St 36)	Together, these points fortify the spleen and
Yin Ling Quan (Sp 9)	percolate dampness.

Chinese medicinal formula: *Shen Ling Bai Zhu San* (Ginseng, Poria & Atractylodes Powder)

Ingredients: Radix Panacis Ginseng (*Ren Shen*), 5g, Sclerotium Poriae Cocos (*Fu Ling*), 12g, Rhizoma Atractylodis Macrocephalae (*Bai Zhu*), 12g, Radix Dioscoreae Oppositae (*Shan Yao*), 10g, Semen Coicis Lachryma-jobi (*Yi Yi Ren*), 20g, Semen Dolichoris Lablab (*Bai Bian Dou*), 10g, Semen Nelumbinis Nuciferae (*Lian Zi*), 10g, Fructus Amomi (*Sha Ren*), 6g, Radix Platycodi Grandiflori (*Jie Geng*), 6g, mix-fried Radix Glycyrrhizae (*Zhi Gan Cao*), 3g

4. Yang vacuity of the spleen & kidneys

Symptoms: Vacuous swelling of the eyelids with drained white skin looking like a ball, in some cases, facial swelling can be present, low back and knee pain and weakness, fatigue, lack of strength, and a deep, fine pulse

Therapeutic principles: Warm and supplement the spleen and kidneys

Acupuncture & moxibustion:

Qi Hai (CV 6)	With moxibustion, helps yang to transform qi
Shui Fen (CV 9)	and, combined with *Shui Fen,* disinhibits water
Shui Quan (Ki 5)	Together, these points disinhibit water through
Yin Ling Quan (Sp 9)	urination.
Shen Shu (Bl 23)	Together, with moxibustion, these points warm
Pi Shu (Bl 20)	and supplement the spleen and kidneys.

Chinese medicinal formula: *Shen Qi Wan* (Kidney Qi Pills)

Ingredients: Prepared Radix Rehmanniae (*Shu Di*), 10g, Fructus Corni Officinalis (*Shan Zhu Yu),* 10g, Radix Dioscoreae Oppositae (*Shan Yao*), 6g, Rhizoma Alismatis (*Ze Xie*), 12g, Cortex Radicis Moutan (*Dan Pi*), 6g, Sclerotium Poriae Cocos (*Fu Ling*), 12g, Cortex Cinnamomi Cassiae (*Rou Gui*), 3g, Radix Lateralis Praeparatus Aconiti Carmichaeli (*Fu Zi*), 6g

5. Dual vacuity of the heart & spleen

Symptoms: Soft, vacuous swelling of the eyelids, fatigue, lack of strength, scant food intake, insomnia, heart palpitations or racing of the heart, impaired memory, a pale tongue, and a fine, weak pulse

Therapeutic principles: Fortify the spleen and nourish the heart

Acupuncture & moxibustion: For this pattern of swollen eyelids, acupuncture and moxibustion are not particularly effective.

Chinese medicinal formula: *Gui Pi Tang* (Return the Spleen Decoction)

Ingredients: Rhizoma Atractylodis Macrocephalae (*Bai Zhu*), 10g, Sclerotium Poriae Cocos (*Fu Ling*), 12g, Radix Astragali Membranacei (*Huang Qi*), 12g, Radix Panacis Ginseng (*Ren Shen*), 3g, mix-fried Radix Glycyrrhizae (*Zhi Gan Cao*), 3g, Radix Angelicae Sinensis (*Dang Gui*), 10g, Radix Auklandiae Lappae (*Mu Xiang*), 6g, Radix Polygalae Tenuifoliae (*Yuan Zhi*), 6g, Arillus Euphoriae Longanae (*Long Yan Rou*), 10g, Semen Zizyphi Spinosae (*Suan Zao Ren*), 10g

6
Drooping Upper Eyelid *(Shang Bao Xia Chui)*

This refers to drooping of the upper eyelid which cannot be lifted up properly. Thus the eye is always partially closed in minor cases and totally closed in severe cases. Hence the vision is obstructed. Blepharoptosis, its Western medical name, can be congenital or acquired. Congenital blepharoptosis from heredity and agenesis usually affects both eyes, while blepharoptosis after disease or trauma often affects only one eye. Blepharoptosis secondary to brain problems and orbital tumors is not included herein. This disease seems to be more common in China than in the West and is seen expecially in the elderly.

Disease causes, disease mechanisms:

I. Center qi fall

Center qi fall may be the result of dietary irregularity or constitutional vacuity of the spleen and stomach. With center qi fall, first, there must be spleen qi vacuity. The spleen governs the muscles. When the spleen is vacuous, less qi and blood will be engendered and transformed. Thus the muscles and sinews will not be sufficiently nourished and lack strength. Secondly, center qi is responsible for upbearing and lifting. With center qi fall, this function of upbearing and lifting is affected. Therefore, drooping of the eyelids may follow.

2. Externally contracted wind evils

"Wind is a yang evil and tends to attack the upper part of the body." If wind evils attack the head, remain in the eyelid, and block the network vessels there, qi flow and blood movement will not be as free as they should be. Under such conditions, the sinews and muscles will lose nourishment and finally blepharoptosis may follow.

3. Qi stagnation & blood stasis

In this case, the cause is often qi stagnation and blood stasis due to trauma to the region of the eyes and head. In traumatic injuries, if the sinews are damaged or if the eyelids lose their nourishment due to qi stagnation and blood stasis from the trauma, the eyelid will become slack and blepharoptosis may occur.

Treatment based on pattern discrimination:

I. Center qi fall

Symptoms: Gradual onset and slow exacerbation of eyelid droop, in some cases, less severe drooping in the morning and more severe in the afternoon. In severe cases, drooping closes the eyes entirely. In that case, the patient cannot see through the eyes unless they lift the eyelid with their hand or tilt the head backward to make lifting the eyelid easier. Other symptoms include a weak constitution, a cold body, shortness of breath, lack of strength in the limbs, a pale and tender tongue, and a weak, deep, faint pulse.

Therapeutic principles: Upbear yang and boost the qi

Acupuncture & moxibustion:

Yang Bai (GB 14)	Together, these points move the qi, quicken the
Zan Zhu (Bl 2)	blood, and open the network vessels to lift up the
Yu Yao (M-HN-6)	eyelid.
Tong Zi Liao (GB 1)	
Si Zhu Kong (TB 23)	
Shang Xing (GV 23)	Together, these points upbear the qi to warm and
Bai Hui (GV 20)	nourish the sinews in the eyelids.

Qi Hai (CV 6) *Ming Men* (GV 4)	Together, these points supplement the source qi.
Zu San Li (St 36) *Wei Shu* (Bl 21) *Pi Shu* (Bl 20)	Together, these points fortify the spleen to promote the source of engendering and transforming.

Note: Five or 6 points should be selected from the above for each treatment. Moxibustion can be applied to *Bai Hui, Qi Hai,* and *Ming Men.* When needling the points *Shang Xing* and *Bai Hui,* the needles should be directed in line with the flow of their channels. In each point, the manipulation should last 30 seconds with subsequent needle retention for 20 minutes. Treat 1 time each day with 10 treatments equaling 1 course of treatment.

Chinese medicinal formula: *Bu Zhong Yi Qi Tang* (Supplement the Center & Boost the Qi Decoction)

Ingredients: Radix Astragali Membranacei (*Huang Qi*), 15g, Rhizoma Atractylodis Macrocephalae (*Bai Zhu*), 10g, Radix Panacis Ginseng (*Ren Shen*), 6g, Radix Bupleuri (*Chai Hu*), 3g, Rhizoma Cimicifugae (*Sheng Ma*), 3g, Radix Angelicae Sinensis (*Dang Gui*), 6g, Pericarpium Citri Reticulatae (*Chen Pi*), 10g, mix-fried Radix Glycyrrhizae (*Zhi Gan Cao*), 6g

2. Externally contracted wind evils

Symptoms: Sudden drooping of the eyelid accompanied by itchy eyes, headache with eye distention, a red tongue, and a floating, rapid pulse

Therapeutic principles: Dispel wind and open the network vessels

Acupuncture & moxibustion:

Yang Bai (GB 14) *Yu Yao* (M-HN-6) *Zan Zhu* (Bl 2)	Together, these points move the qi, quicken the blood, and open the network vessels to uplift the eyelid. *(Point list continues on next page.)*

Tong Zi Liao (GB 1)
Si Zhu Kong (TB 23)

Shang Xing (GV 23) *Bai Hui* (GV 20)	Together, these points upbear the qi to warm and nourish the sinews in the eyelids.
Feng Chi (GB 20) *He Gu* (LI 4)	Together, these points course wind.

Note: In each treatment, select 5-6 points from the above. Moxibustion can be applied to *Bai Hui*. In needling the points *Shang Xing* and *Bai Hui,* the needles should be directed in line with the flow of their channels. Each point should be manipulated for 30 seconds with subsequent needle retention for 20 minutes. Treat 1 time each day with 10 treatments equaling 1 course of treatment.

Chinese medicinal formula: *Chu Feng Yi Sun Tang* (Eliminate Wind, Boost & Reduce Decoction)

Ingredients: Radix Ledebouriellae Divaricatae (*Fang Feng*), 12g, Radix Ligustici Wallichii (*Chuan Xiong*), 12g, Radix Peucedani (*Qian Hu*), 10g, Radix Et Rhizoma Ligustici Chinensis (*Gao Ben*), 12g, Radix Albus Paeoniae Lactiflorae (*Bai Shao*), 6g, Radix Angelicae Sinensis (*Dang Gui*), 9g, prepared Radix Rehmanniae (*Shu Di*), 9g

3. Qi stagnation & blood stasis

Symptoms: A history of trauma to the eyes or head. If the trauma happened recently, swelling and pain may be present in addition to the main complaint of eyelid drooping. Other concomitant symptoms are seldom seen.

Therapeutic principles: Move the qi and quicken the blood

Acupuncture & moxibustion:

Yang Bai (GB 14) *Zan Zhu* (Bl 2) *Yu Yao* (M-HN-6) *Tong Zi Liao* (GB 1) *Si Zhu Kong* (TB 23)	Together, these points move the qi, quicken the blood, and open the network vessels to uplift the eyelid.
Shang Xing (GV 23) *Bai Hui* (GV 20)	Together, these points upbear the qi to warm and nourish the sinews of the eyelids.
San Yin Jiao (Sp 6) *He Gu* (LI 4)	Together, these points move the qi and quicken the blood.

Note: Select 5-6 points each treatment from the above. Moxibustion can be applied to *Bai Hui.* When needling the points *Shang Xing* and *Bai Hui,* the needles should be directed in line with the flow of their channels. Manipulate each point for 30 seconds with subsequent needle retention for 20 minutes. Treat 1 time each day with 10 treatments equaling 1 course of treatment.

Chinese medicinal formula: *Qu Yu Si Wu Tang* (Dispel Stasis Four Materials Decoction)

Ingredients: Radix Angelicae Sinensis (*Dang Gui*), 12g, Radix Rubrus Paeoniae Lactiflorae (*Chi Shao*), 12g, Radix Ligustici Wallichii (*Chuan Xiong*), 12g, Herba Leonuri Heterophylli (*Yi Mu Cao*), 15g, Flos Carthami Tinctorii (*Hong Hua*), 6g, Radix Artemisiae Anomalae (*Liu Ji Nu*), 9g

7
Phlegm Pit in the Eyelid *(Bao Sheng Tan He)*

Phlegm pit in the eyelid refers to a round, hard, painless mass in the eyelid. This is seen more in the upper lid than in the lower. This traditional Chinese disease category covers hordeolum or sty as well as chalazion in Western medicine.

Disease causes, disease mechanisms:

I. Phlegm dampness accumulation & binding

Accumulation and binding of phlegm dampness may arise from spleen vacuity due to dietary irregularity, constitutional spleen yang vacuity, etc. With impairment of spleen movement and transformation, water dampness may accumulate internally, and, over time, this may transform into phlegm dampness. If this phlegm dampness flows upward and stagnates in the network vessels of the eyelids, little by little, it will bind with qi and blood passing by and, therefore, a mass in the eyelid is formed.

2. Phlegm & fire combining

Addiction to alcohol and fatty or spicy food may first of all damage the spleen and stomach and cause the accumulation of dampness in the center due to impairment of spleen movement and transformation. Secondly, heat will be engendered. If dampness and heat bind with each other and brew in the spleen and stomach, phlegm fire may be formed. Because phlegm is liquid-like in form, it can flow. If phlegm binds with fire and then flows up to and stagnates in the network vessels, it may further combine with the qi and blood passing by. Therefore, a mass in the eyelid may occur.

Treatment based on pattern discrimination:

I. Phlegm dampness accumulation & binding

Symptoms: There is a painless, hard, visible, and palpable mass under the skin of the eyelid. The size can vary from that of a grain of rice to a broad bean. No pain or itching is present. The skin, which is normal in color, can be moved loosely over the swelling, which may also be seen in the tarsus of the lid. The patient may feel heaviness and distention in the lid and a slight sensation of a foreign body in the eye if the mass reaches a certain size. No obvious systemic symptoms can be observed.

Therapeutic principles: Transform phlegm, soften hardness, and scatter nodulation

Acupuncture & moxibustion: Based on the authors' knowledge and experience, acupuncture and moxibustion do not work very well for chalazion.

Chinese medicinal formula: Modified *Hua Jian Er Chen Wan* (Transform Hardness Two Aged [Ingredients] Decoction)

Ingredients: Rhizoma Pinelliae Ternatae (*Ban Xia*), 12g, Pericarpium Citri Reticulatae (*Chen Pi*), 12g, Sclerotium Poriae Cocos (*Fu Ling*), 12g, Bombyx Batryticatus (*Jiang Can*), 10g, Folium Nelumbinis Nuciferae (*He Ye*), 10g, Radix Scrophulariae Ningpoensis (*Xuan Shen*), 10g

2. Phlegm & fire combining

Symptoms: Pain, itching, and swelling of the eyelid is the main complaint. The local skin is slightly red above the swelling, which may be seen in the tarsus of the lid. This generally presents subconjunctivally as a red or purple mass. Other symptoms include a dry mouth and throat, a red tongue, and a rapid pulse

Therapeutic principles: Transform phlegm, clear heat, and scatter nodulation

Acupuncture & moxibustion: Again, acupuncture and moxibustion do not work very well for chalazion.

Chinese medicinal formula: Modified *Qing Wei Tang* (Clear Stomach Decoction)

Ingredients: Gypsum Fibrosum (*Shi Gao*), 15g, Radix Scutellariae Baicalensis (*Huang Qin*), 6g, Rhizoma Coptidis Chinensis (*Huang Lian*), 6g, uncooked Radix Rehmanniae (*Sheng Di*), 10g, Cortex Radicis Moutan (*Dan Pi*), 10g, uncooked Rhizoma Cimicifugae (*Sheng Ma*), 6g, Radix Scrophulariae Ningpoensis (*Xuan Shen*), 10g, Rhizoma Pinelliae Ternatae (*Ban Xia*), 10g, Bombyx Batryticatus (*Jiang Can*), 10g

8
Orbital Pain *(Yan Kuang Tong)*

This refers to a feeling of aching and pain around the orbit of the eye with possible heaviness of the eyelids and photophobia. It often occurs along with headache.

Disease causes, disease mechanisms:

I. Externally contracted wind cold

The *tai yang* channel is the fence of the body. When wind cold invades the body, very often the *tai yang* channel is the first to be affected. If externally contracted wind cold goes upward along the *tai yang* channel to the ligation of the eye, obstruction may occur in the network vessels since cold evils by nature are contracting. This can then prevent the qi and blood from flowing freely. With obstruction or stagnation in that area, orbital pain may occur. This is based on the saying, "Where there is no free flow, there is pain."

2. Yin vacuity & yang hyperactivity

Yin vacuity and yang hyperactivity may arise from blood loss, severe disease, postpartum, sexual taxation, etc. With yin vacuity, yang, and especially liver yang, will become hyperactive. This is because, in the liver, "Yang often is surplus, while yin is commonly insufficient." The liver channel connects with the ligation of the eye. If ascendent liver yang goes along this channel and harasses the head and eyes, pain may occur in the orbit of the eye.

Treatment based on pattern discrimination:

I. Externally contracted wind cold

Symptoms: Aversion to cold with fever, fear of wind, distended pain in the eyes and head, aching in the orbit, aching in the joints, thin, white tongue fur, and a floating, tight pulse

Therapeutic principles: Course wind, dissipate cold, and stop pain

Acupuncture & moxibustion:

Feng Chi (GB 20)	Together, these points course wind and scatter cold
Zan Zhu (Bl 2)	to stop pain.
Yang Bai (GB 14)	

He Gu (LI 4)	Together, these points course wind and scatter cold.
Wai Guan (TB 5)	

Note: When needling the point *Zan Zhu,* the needle should be inserted transversely from medial to lateral along the eyebrow.

Chinese medicinal formula: *Chuan Xiong Cha Tiao San* (Ligusticum Wallichium & Tea Regulating Powder)

Ingredients: Herba Cum Radice Asari (*Xi Xin*), 3g, Radix Ligustici Wallichii (*Chuan Xiong*), 12g, Radix Et Rhizoma Notopterygii (*Qiang Huo*), 10g, Radix Ledebouriellae Divaricatae (*Fang Feng*), 10g, Herba Schizonepetae Tenuifoliae (*Jing Jie*), 10g, Herba Menthae Haplocalycis (*Bo He*), 3g, Radix Angelicae Dahuricae (*Bai Zhi*), 10g, Radix Glycyrrhizae (*Gan Cao*), 3g

2. Yin vacuity & yang hyperactivity

Symptoms: Aching pain in the orbit, headache, especially in the temple, dizziness, heaviness of the eyelids, photophobia, vexation and agitation, irascibility, tinnitus, insomnia, a dry mouth, a red face, a red tongue with scant or thin, yellow fur, and a wiry, fine, and rapid pulse

Therapeutic principles: Level the liver and subdue yang

Acupuncture & moxibustion:

Tou Ling Qi (GB 15)	Together, these points help subdue yang and
Si Zhu Kong (TB 23)	harmonize the network vessels to stop pain.
Zan Zhu (Bl 2)	

Tai Chong (Liv 3)	Together, these points level the liver and subdue
Tai Xi (Ki 3)	yang.
Xing Jian (Liv 2)	

Chinese medicinal formula: *Tian Ma Gou Teng Yin* (Gastrodia & Uncaria Drink)

Ingredients: Rhizoma Gastrodiae Elatae (*Tian Ma*), 10g, Ramulus Uncariae Cum Uncis (*Gou Teng*), 10g, Cortex Eucommiae Ulmoidis (*Du Zhong*), 10g, Radix Achyranthis Bidentatae (*Huai Niu Xi*), 10g, Concha Haliotidis (*Shi Jue Ming*), 15g, Ramulus Loranthi Seu Visci (*Sang Ji Sheng*), 10g, Fructus Gardeniae Jasminoidis (*Zhi Zi*), 6g, Radix Scutellariae Baicalensis (*Huang Qin*), 6g, Herba Leonuri Heterophylli (*Yi Mu Cao*), 15g, Caulis Polygoni Multiflori (*Ye Jiao Teng*), 6g, Sclerotium Pararadicis Poriae Cocos (*Fu Shen*), 6g

9
Tearing in the Wind *(Ying Feng Liu Lei)*

Tearing in the wind refers to persistent tearing of the eyes which is precipitated or exacerbated by wind. Tearing secondary to other eye diseases or from injury is not dealt with herein.

Disease causes, disease mechanisms:

I. Wind heat in the liver channel

Constitutional exuberance of yang or emotional disturbance, such as anger and frustration, may lead to heat brewing in the liver channel. In this case, external wind evils may take advantage of this to invade the body and combine easily with the heat brewing in the liver channel. When heat and wind in combination attack upward to the eyes along the channel, the qi dynamic in the network vessels of the eyes will be inhibited and the flow of the "humor of the liver," *i.e.*, the tears, may be affected. Hence there is tearing.

2. Yin vacuity, fire effulgence

Overthinking often can consume heart blood surreptitiously. Heart fire is the son of liver wood, and heart blood vacuity will lead to liver blood vacuity over time. In the long run, liver/kidney yin will also be rendered vacuous, since "The liver and kidneys share a common source." Yin/blood vacuity of the liver and kidneys will thus typically bring about yin vacuity fire which may flame upward. When this fire disturbs the flow of the "humor of the liver," there will be tearing.

3. Liver blood vacuity

Liver blood vacuity may come from great loss of blood, chronic disease, spleen/stomach vacuity, heart blood vacuity, or aging. With liver blood vacuity, the portals of the eyes will not be nourished sufficiently and thus the eyes become susceptible to invasion by external wind cold. Cold by its very nature leads to contraction of the network vessels of the eyes, and hence the flow of the "humor of the liver" will be affected. As a result, tearing may occur.

4. Dual vacuity of the liver & kidneys

Sexual intemperance, aging, or profuse crying due to grief may lead to yin vacuity of the liver and kidneys. Over time, this yin vacuity will render yang vacuous as well. When there is yang vacuity, the network vessels of the eyes will not be properly warmed and thus the flow of the "humor of the liver" will not be contained. This is because yang qi is responsible for warming and containing. Thus, when there is dual vacuity of the liver and kidneys, there may also be tearing.

Treatment based on pattern discrimination

I. Wind heat in the liver channel

Symptoms: Hot tearing in the wind, redness of the eyes, a rough sensation in eyes, a dry mouth and throat, dizziness, tinnitus, a red tongue with thin, white fur, and a wiry, fine, rapid pulse

Therapeutic principles: Clear the liver, dispel wind, and stop tearing

Acupuncture & moxibustion:

Jing Ming (Bl 1)	Together, these points regulate the qi and blood
Zan Zhu (Bl 2)	locally to promote the flow of the "humor of the
Cheng Qi (St 1)	liver" and stop tearing.

He Gu (LI 4) With draining method, dissipates wind heat

Tai Chong (Liv 3) Together, with draining method, these points clear
Yang Bai (GB 14) and drain heat in liver/gallbladder.

Additions & subtractions: If wind heat is predominant, add *Wai Guan* (TB 5). If liver fire is predominant, add *Xia Xi* (GB 43) and *Yang Fu* (GB 38). If there is simultaneous headache, add *Shen Ting* (GV 24).

Remarks: Acupuncture is effective for this type of tearing. However, the rules on needle insertion and manipulation for the local points should be carefully observed.

Chinese medicinal formula: Modified *Ling Yang Jiao San* (Antelope Horn Powder)

Ingredients: Cornu Caprae (*Shan Yang Jiao*), 10g, Radix Et Rhizoma Notopterygii (*Qiang Huo*), 10g, Radix Scrophulariae Ningpoensis (*Xuan Shen*), 10g, Semen Plantaginis (*Che Qian Zi*), 12g, Fructus Gardeniae Jasminoidis (*Zhi Zi*), 6g, Radix Scutellariae Baicalensis (*Huang Qin*), 6g, Fructus Viticis (*Man Jing Zi*), 10g, Flos Chrysanthemi Morifolii (*Ju Hua*), 12g, Herba Equiseti Hiemalis (*Mu Zei*), 10g, Spica Prunellae Vulgaris (*Xia Ku Cao*), 10g

Note: The name of this formula is *Ling Yang Jiao San* (Antelope Horn Powder) but its first ingredient is Cornu Caprae (*Shan Yang Jiao*) or goat horn. This substitution is because the Saiga Antelope from which Cornu Antelopis Saiga-tatarici comes is an endangered species.

2. Yin vacuity, fire effulgence

Symptoms: Hot tearing during the day with dry eyes at night, dizziness, clouded vision, a red tongue with thin or thin, yellow fur, and a fine, rapid pulse

Therapeutic principles: Enrich and supplement the liver and kidneys and stop tearing

Acupuncture & moxibustion:

Jing Ming (Bl 1)   Together, these points regulate the qi and blood
Zan Zhu (Bl 2)   locally to promote the flow of the "humor of the
Tou Ling Qi (GB 15) liver" and stop tearing.

Tai Chong (Liv 3) Together, these points subdue effulgent fire due to
Tai Xi (Ki 3)   yin vacuity. Drain *Tai Chong* and supplement *Tai Xi*.

Additions & subtractions: If there is blurred vision, add *Yang Lao* (SI 6).

Chinese medicinal formula: Modified *Qi Ju Di Huang Wan* (Lycium & Chrysanthemum Rehmannia Pills)

Ingredients: Prepared Radix Rehmanniae (*Shu Di*), 10g, Fructus Corni Officinalis (*Shan Zhu Yu*), 10g, Radix Dioscoreae Oppositae (*Shan Yao*), 10g, Semen Plantaginis (*Che Qian Zi*), 12g, Cortex Radicis Moutan (*Dan Pi*), 10g, Sclerotium Poriae Cocos (*Fu Ling*), 6g, Fructus Lycii Chinensis (*Gou Qi Zi*), 12g, Flos Chrysanthemi Morifolii (*Ju Hua*), 12g, Fructus Ligustri Lucidi (*Nu Zhen Zi*), 12g

Additions & subtractions: If there are symptoms from liver fire, replace prepared Radix Rehmanniae (*Shu Di*) with uncooked Radix Rehmanniae (*Sheng Di*), subtract Sclerotium Poriae Cocos (*Fu Ling*), and add Spica Prunellae Vulgaris (*Xia Ku Cao*), 10g, Semen Cassiae Torae (*Jue Ming Zi*), 15g.

3. Liver blood vacuity

Symptoms: Cold tearing in the wind, emaciation, a sallow yellow facial complexion, pale lips and nails, a pale tongue, and a fine pulse. In severe cases, one may see cold limbs, a pale tongue with moist, white fur, and a deep, slow pulse.

Therapeutic principles: Nourish the blood, dispel cold, and stop tearing

Acupuncture & moxibustion:

Jing Ming (Bl 1) *Cheng Qi* (St 1)	Together, these points regulate the flow of the "humor of the liver" to stop tearing. Do not manipulate these points.
Feng Chi (GB 20)	With draining method, dispels cold and opens the network vessels in the eyes
San Yin Jiao (Sp 6)	With supplementing technique for 1 minute, helps engender the blood

Additions & subtractions: If there is blurred vision, add *Yang Lao* (SI 6).

Chinese medicinal formula: Modified *Yang Xue Qu Han Yin* (Nourish the Blood & Dispel Cold Drink)

Ingredients: Radix Angelicae Sinensis (*Dang Gui*), 12g, Fructus Lycii Chinensis (*Gou Qi Zi*), 12g, Fructus Rubi Chingii (*Fu Pen Zi*), 12g, Flos Chrysanthemi Morifolii (*Ju Hua*), 12g, Rhizoma Atractylodis (*Cang Zhu*), 10g, Radix Albus Paeoniae Lactiflorae (*Bai Shao*), 10g, Rhizoma Atractylodis Macrocephalae (*Bai Zhu*), 6g, Sclerotium Poriae Cocos (*Fu Ling*), 6g, Radix Ligustici Wallichii (*Chuan Xiong*), 6g, Cortex Cinnamomi Cassiae (*Rou Gui*), 3g, Herba Cum Radice Asari (*Xi Xin*), 3g

Additions & subtractions: If there is blurred vision from endured tearing, prescribe Modified *Gou Qi Zi Jiu* (Lycium Wine).

Ingredients: Fructus Lycii Chinensis (*Gou Qi Zi*), 30g, Fructus Ligustri Lucidi (*Nu Zhen Zi*), 30g, Fructus Mori Albi (*Sang Shen*), 30g, rice wine

(*Huang Jiu*), 300ml. Steep these medicinals in the rice wine for 2 weeks to 1 month. Then remove the dregs and store for use. Drink 10ml each time, 2 times each day.

4. Dual vacuity of the liver & kidneys

Symptoms: Persistent cold tearing which is exacerbated by exposure to cold, vertigo, blurred vision, tinnitus or deafness, insomnia, seminal emission, low back and knee pain and weakness, white tongue fur, and a fine, weak pulse

Therapeutic principles: Warm and nourish the liver and kidneys, supplement and boost the essence and blood, stop tearing

Acupuncture & moxibustion:

Jing Ming (Bl 1) *Zan Zhu* (Bl 2)	Together, these points promote the flow of the "humor of the liver" to stop tearing.
Gan Shu (Bl 18) *Feng Chi* (GB 20) *Pi Shu* (Bl 20) *Shen Shu* (Bl 23)	Together, these points supplement the liver, boost the kidneys, and fortify the spleen to contain "the humor of the liver." Apply moxibustion to the handle of the needles.

Additions & subtractions: If there is headache, add *Tou Ling Qi* (GB 15).

Remarks: Acupuncture and moxibustion are not very effective when used alone for this pattern of tearing but can be used as adjunctive therapy along with internally administered Chinese medicinals.

Chinese medicinal formula: Modified *Ju Jing Wan* (Chrysanthemum Eye Pills)

Ingredients: Flos Chrysanthemi Morifolii (*Ju Hua*), 10g, Radix Morindae Officinalis (*Ba Ji Tian*), 10g, Herba Cistanchis Deserticolae (*Rou Cong Rong*), 10g, Fructus Lycii Chinensis (*Gou Qi Zi*), 12g, Semen Cuscutae Chinensis (*Tu Si Zi*), 12g, Semen Astragali Complanati (*Sha Yuan Zi*), 10g

10
Photophobia & Pyretophobia of the Eyes
(Xiu Ming Pa Re)

Photophobia refers to pain, discomfort, or a rough sensation of the eyes or difficulty opening the eyes when exposed to bright light. Pyretophobia means pain or discomfort of the eyes due to exposure to warmth.

Disease causes, disease mechanisms:

The eyes collect essence and qi from all five viscera. When supported by sufficient essence and qi from the five viscera, the eyes can see accurately and can withstand normal external stimulation without problem. Thus, if the eyes fail to obtain sufficient nourishment due to vacuity or if evils cause blockage in the network vessels of the eyes, photophobia and pyretophobia may occur. In clinic, the following patterns are the most commonly seen.

1. Wind cold fettering the exterior

When wind cold attacks the body, the defensive qi will be affected and disharmony of the defensive qi will occur. Then the lung qi will become depressed and stagnant. The whites of the eyes are made from lung essence. When lung qi is depressed and stagnant, the network vessels in the whites of the eyes will become blocked. As a result, there is less nourishment to support the eyes. Therefore, the eyes cannot stand light and warmth as they should do, and photophobia and pyretophobia may occur.

2. Qi vacuity & wind heat invasion

Qi vacuity may be due prenatally to insufficient natural endowment and postnatally to poor nourishment, chronic disease, aging, or taxation. If the qi is vacuous, first, the essence and blood cannot be moved to nourish the eyes. Secondly, the body will become susceptible to invasion by external evils. If wind heat takes advantage of vacuity to invade the body and attacks the portals of the eyes, blockage may result in the eyes and thus the nourishment of the eyes will deteriorate. Consequently photophobia and pyretophobia may occur.

3. Dual vacuity of the qi & yin

Qi and yin vacuity may arise from congenital insufficiency, aging, chronic diseases, sexual taxation, etc. With dual vacuity of the qi and yin, first, there will be less nourishment supplied to the eyes. Secondly, yin vacuity fire may counterflow upward to disturb the qi and blood in the eyes, causing disharmony of the qi and blood in that region. In this case, the nourishment in the eyes will become even worse. Thus photophobia and pyretophobia may occur.

Treatment based on pattern discrimination:

I. Wind cold fettering the exterior

Symptoms: Red eyes with slight pain, a rough sensation in the eyes, profuse, sticky eye discharge, photophobia, pyretophobia, stuck together eyelashes, swelling at the inner ends of the eyebrow, aversion to wind and cold, nasal congestion, runny nose, thin, white tongue fur, and a floating, tight pulse

Therapeutic principles: Course wind, scatter cold, and resolve the exterior, quicken the blood and move stasis

Acupuncture & moxibustion:

Zan Zhu (Bl 2)	Together, with draining method, these points
Yu Yao (M-HN-6)	course and free the network vessels in the eyes.

Feng Chi (GB 20)   A point on the gallbladder channel which is very effective for eye problems. Here, it courses wind and dissipates cold in the head and eyes.

He Gu (LI 4)   The source point of the hand *yang ming* channel

Wai Guan (TB 5)   The network of the triple burner and a meeting point of the eight vessels
Together, these points can invigorate yang to course wind and scatter cold.

Chinese medicinal formula: Modified *Ming Mu Xi Xin Tang* (Brighten the Eyes Asarum Decoction)

Ingredients: Herba Cum Radice Asari (*Xi Xin*), 3g, Radix Ledebouriellae Divaricatae (*Fang Feng*), 10g, Radix Et Rhizoma Notopterygii (*Qiang Huo*), 10g, Herba Schizonepetae Tenuifoliae (*Jing Jie*), 10g, Radix Ligustici Wallichii (*Chuan Xiong*), 10g, Radix Et Rhizoma Ligustici Chinensis (*Gao Ben*), 10g, Herba Ephedrae (*Ma Huang*), 6g, Pericarpium Zanthoxyli Bungeani (*Hua Jiao*), 3g, Radix Angelicae Sinensis (*Dang Gui*), 6g, Flos Carthami Tinctorii (*Hong Hua*), 6g, Semen Pruni Persicae (*Tao Ren*), 6g, Fructus Viticis (*Man Jing Zi*), 10g

2. Qi vacuity & wind heat invasion

Symptoms: Tightness in the canthus, photophobia, pyretophobia, tearing in the wind, blurred vision on lengthy looking, a pale tongue, and a fine, rapid pulse

Therapeutic principles: Boost the qi and support the correct, course wind and clear heat

Acupuncture & moxibustion:

Zan Zhu (Bl 2) *Feng Chi* (GB 20) *Si Zhu Kong* (TB 23)	Together, these points dispel wind, clear heat, and open the network vessels in the eyes.
Bai Hui (GV 20)	Upbears essence and qi from the five viscera to nourish the eye
Qi Hai (CV 6) *Yuan* (CV 4)	Key points to boost the qi and help upbear *Guan* essence of the five viscera to nourish the eyes so as to withstand light and warmth

Chinese medicinal formula: *Lian Qiao Yin Zi* (Forsythia Drink)

Ingredients: Fructus Forsythiae Suspensae (*Lian Qiao*), 10g, Radix Angelicae Sinensis (*Dang Gui*), 10g, Radix Panacis Ginseng (*Ren Shen*), 5g, mix-fried Radix Glycyrrhizae (*Zhi Gan Cao*), 6g, Radix Astragali Membranacei (*Huang Qi*), 12g, Fructus Viticis (*Man Jing Zi*), 10g, uncooked Radix Rehmanniae (*Sheng Di*), 6g, Rhizoma Cimicifugae (*Sheng Ma*), 6g, Radix Scutellariae Baicalensis (*Huang Qin*), 6g, Radix Et Rhizoma Notopterygii (*Qiang Huo*), 10g, Radix Bupleuri (*Chai Hu*), 6g

3. Dual vacuity of the qi & yin

Symptoms: Photophobia and pyretophobia, blurred vision, inclination to close the eyes, slightly sore, red whites of the eyes, dizziness, tinnitus, a dry mouth and throat, possible loose stools and fear of cold in the lower limbs, thin, white tongue fur, and a fine pulse

Therapeutic principles: Boost the qi and nourish yin, clear heat and subdue fire. If there is yang vacuity, boost the qi and warm yang.

Acupuncture & moxibustion:

Jing Ming (Bl 1)	Together, these points harmonize the qi and
Zan Zhu (Bl 2)	blood in the eyes.
Bai Hui (GV 20)	Upbears the qi and essence to nourish the eyes
Ming Men (CV 4)	Together, these points boost the qi and yin to
Shen Shu (Bl 23)	nourish the eyes and help the eyes to withstand
Guan Yuan (CV 4)	light and warmth.

Note: When yang vacuity is obvious, moxibustion should be applied to the needle handles at *Bai Hui*, *Guan Yuan*, *Shen Shu,* and *Ming Men*.

Remarks: In the treatment of photophobia and pyretophobia, acupuncture and moxibustion are not as effective as internal Chinese medicine. It is, therefore, advisable to use acupuncture and moxibustion in combination with other such therapies when treating these conditions.

Chinese medicinal formula: *Zi Yin Di Huang Wan* (Enrich Yin Rehmannia Pills)

Ingredients: Prepared Radix Rehmanniae (*Shu Di*), 12g, Radix Dioscoreae Oppositae (*Shan Yao*), 10g, Fructus Corni Officinalis (*Shan Zhu Yu*), 10g, Fructus Schisandrae Chinensis (*Wu Wei Zi*), 10g, Tuber Ophiopogonis Japonici (*Mai Dong*), 10g, Radix Angelicae Sinensis (*Dang Gui*), 10g, Flos Chrysanthemi Morifolii (*Ju Hua*), 12g, Fructus Lycii Chinensis (*Gou Qi Zi*), 12g, Herba Cistanchis Deserticolae (*Rou Cong Rong*), 10g, Radix Morindae Officinalis (*Ba Ji Tian*), 10g.

Additions & subtractions: If there is dual vacuity of yin and yang, add Cortex Cinnamomi Cassiae (*Rou Gui*), 3g, Semen Astragali Complanati (*Sha Yuan Zi*), 10g, and Semen Cuscutae Chinensis (*Tu Si Zi*), 10g. If there is vacuity heat, add Rhizoma Anemarrhenae Asphodeloidis (*Zhi Mu*), 10g, and Cortex Phellodendri (*Huang Bai*), 10g

II
Reddening of the Eyes *(Mu Chi)*

Reddening of the eyes means that the whites of the eyes become red in color. This may occur in one or both of the eyes.

Disease causes, disease mechanisms:

I. Externally contracted wind heat

Patients with constitutional exuberant yang are more susceptible to contraction of external wind heat. If wind and heat invade the body in combination and attack the eyes, the body's correct qi will struggle with the wind and heat in the eyes. As a result, the qi and blood stagnate in the network vessels of the eyes, and, therefore, reddening of the eyes may occur. On the other hand, if heat is predominant, it may burn the network vessels and the blood will then flow outside of the vessels. As a result, the whites of the eyes will become red as well.

2. Epidemic qi

Patients with heat accumulation in the lungs or stomach are liable to be infected by epidemic qi. If the epidemic qi attacks the eyes in combination with this accumulated heat, the flow of qi and blood in the eyes will be disturbed. Stagnation of qi and blood in the eyes will then lead to reddening of the eyes.

3. Heat evils deep-lying in the network vessels

"In enduring disease, evils enter the network vessels." Therefore, it is common that an enduring hot eye disease may leave heat evils lingering in the network vessels in the eyes. In addition, an enduring exposure to wind with dust, fire, smoke, or addiction to strong alcoholic beverages, toasted and spicy foods, or enduring taxation of the eyesight may all lead to heat evils deep-lying in the network vessels. When pathogens lie deeply in the network vessels in the eyes, the flow of qi and blood there will stagnate and, therefore, reddening of the eyes may occur.

4. Alcohol toxins brewing internally

An enduring addiction to alcoholic beverages may damage the spleen and lead to alcohol toxins brewing in the interior. With time, heat will accumulate. Because the spleen is damaged, spleen earth will become weaker. At the same time, invaded by the accumulated heat, liver wood will become stronger and overcheck the spleen. With more and more accumulation of heat, heat will tend to counterflow upward along the liver channel to eventually attack the eyes. If alcohol toxins and heat accumulate in the network vessels of the eyes, reddening of the eyes may occur.

5. Exuberant liver/gallbladder fire

Exuberant liver/gallbladder fire may arise from emotional disturbance, such as depression, frustration and anger, externally contracted damp heat, or spleen damage from improper dietary habits. The eyes are the portals of the liver and the liver channel connects with the eyes. If exuberant liver/gallbladder fire attacks the eyes along the channel, the network vessels in the eyes will be burnt and the blood may flow out of the vessels. As a result, reddening of the eyes occurs.

6. Yin vacuity of the liver & kidneys

Yin vacuity of the liver and kidneys may result from congenital insufficiency, chronic disease, aging, sexual taxation, etc. With yin vacuity of the liver and kidneys, vacuity fire may exist. If vacuity fire counterflows upward and attacks the eyes, the flow of qi and blood in the eyes will be disturbed. Therefore, reddening of the eyes may occur.

Treatment based on pattern discrimination:

I. Externally contracted wind heat

Symptoms: During the early stage, there may be sudden reddening of the whites of the eyes, hot tearing, photophobia, and a rough sensation in the eyes. Concomitant symptoms may include aversion to cold, fever, headache, nasal congestion, thin, white tongue fur, and a floating, rapid pulse. In severe cases, pain in the eyeballs may render the patient restless.

Therapeutic principles: Course wind and clear heat

Acupuncture & moxibustion:

Feng Chi (GB 20) A point on the gallbladder channel which has an exterior/interior relationship with the liver channel. This point can course wind and clear heat in the head and the eyes when needled with draining method.

Shang Xing (GV 23) Together, with draining method, these points can
Yu Yao (M-HN-8) open the network vessels in the eyes to free the
Tai Yang (M-HN-9) flow of qi and blood in the eyes.

He Gu (LI 4) The source point of the hand *yang ming* channel; with draining method, it courses wind and clears heat.

Additions & subtractions: *Shang Xing, Tai Yang, Yu Yao,* and *He Gu* should be pricked to induce bleeding in order to clear heat when heat is predominant. The manifestations of this are severe sore, red eyes, sticky eye discharge, thirst, dark urine, yellow tongue fur, and a rapid, replete pulse. If there is constipation, add *Nei Ting* (St 44). If there are concurrent exterior and interior patterns, add *Qu Chi* (LI 11) and *Nei Ting* (St 44).

Chinese medicinal formula: Modified *Qiang Huo Sheng Feng Tang* (Notopterygium Overcome Wind Decoction)

Ingredients: Herba Menthae Haplocalycis (*Bo He*), 6g, Radix Bupleuri (*Chai Hu*), 6g, Radix Scutellariae Baicalensis (*Huang Qin*), 6g, Radix Et Rhizoma Notopterygii (*Qiang Huo*), 10g, Herba Schizonepetae Tenuifoliae (*Jing Jie*), 10g, Radix Ligustici Wallichii (*Chuan Xiong*), 10g, Radix Ledebouriellae Divaricatae (*Fang Feng*), 10g, Fructus Viticis (*Man Jing Zi*), 10g, Radix Angelicae Dahuricae (*Bai Zhi*), 10g, Radix Peucedani (*Qian Hu*), 10g, Herba Equiseti Hiemalis (*Mu Zei*), 10g, Folium Mori Albi (*Sang Ye*), 10g

Additions & subtractions: If there is constipation, add Radix Et Rhizoma Rhei (*Da Huang*), 9g, and Mirabilitum (*Mang Xiao*), 9g.

If heat is predominant: Modified *Xie Fei Yin* (Drain Lung Drink)

Ingredients: Gypsum Fibrosum (*Shi Gao*), 15g, Radix Rubrus Paeoniae Lactiflorae (*Chi Shao*), 10g, Radix Scutellariae Baicalensis (*Huang Qin*), 10g, Folium Mori Albi (*Sang Ye*), 10g, Caulis Akebiae (*Mu Tong*), 5g, Fructus Forsythiae Suspensae (*Lian Qiao*), 10g, Herba Schizonepetae Tenuifolia (*Jing Jie*), 10g, Radix Ledebouriellae Divaricatae (*Fang Feng*), 10g, Radix Angelicae Dahuricae (*Bai Zhi*), 10g, Radix Et Rhizoma Notopterygii (*Qiang Huo*), 10g, Flos Chrysanthemi Morifolii (*Ju Hua*), 12g, Radix Glycyrrhizae (*Gan Cao*), 6g

If there is simultaneous exterior and interior heat: Modified *Ju Hua Tong Shen San* (Chrysanthemum Sagely Opening Powder):

Ingredients: Flos Chrysanthemi Morifolii (*Ju Hua*), 15g, Radix Ledebouriellae Divaricatae (*Fang Feng*), 10g, Radix Et Rhizoma Notopterygii (*Qiang Huo*), 10g, Herba Menthae Haplocalycis (*Bo He*), 6g, Fructus Forsythiae Suspensae (*Lian Qiao*), 10g, Herba Ephedrae (*Ma Huang*), 6g, Herba Schizonepetae Tenuifoliae (*Jing Jie*), 10g, Fructus Gardeniae Jasminoidis (*Zhi Zi*), 6g, Gypsum Fibrosum (*Shi Gao*), 15g,

Radix Scutellariae Baicalensis (*Huang Qin*), 10g, Radix Et Rhizoma Rhei (*Da Huang*), 6g, Mirabilitum (*Mang Xiao*), 6g, Radix Angelicae Sinensis (*Dang Gui*), 6g, Radix Ligustici Wallichii (*Chuan Xiong*), 10g, Rhizoma Coptidis Chinensis (*Huang Lian*), 6g

2. Epidemic qi

Symptoms: Reddening of the whites of the eyes with a burning sensation, sticky eye discharge, photophobia, difficulty in opening the eyes due to a rough sensation in the eyes. In some cases, one eye is affected, and, in other cases, both of the eyes are involved.

Therapeutic principles: Course wind, discharge heat, and resolve toxins

Acupuncture & moxibustion:

Zan Zhu (Bl 2)   Prick the point to let 3-5 drops of blood from each.

Tai Yang (M-HN 9) Pricking the point to bleed resolves toxins, clears heat, and courses wind.

Needle *a shi* points in the region of the eye or in the region of the ear corresponding to the eye.

Additions & subtractions: If there is severe burning pain in the eyes, yellow tongue fur, and a rapid pulse, add *Qu Chi* (LI 11) and *He Gu* (LI 4). Prick to induce bleeding. If there is constipation, add *Nei Ting* (St 44) and *Zhi Gou* (TB 6).

Remarks: The above is a very effective method of treatment for epidemic reddening of the eyes. Better results will be achieved if one also applies proper antibiotic eye drops.

Chinese medicinal formula: Modified *Qu Feng San Re Yin Zi* (Dispel Wind, Dissipate Heat Drink)

Ingredients: Fructus Forsythiae Suspensae (*Lian Qiao*), 12g, Flos Lonicerae Japonicae (*Yin Hua*), 15g, Fructus Arctii Lappae (*Niu Bang Zi*), 10g, Herba Menthae Haplocalycis (*Bo He*), 6g, Fructus Gardeniae Jasminoidis (*Zhi Zi*), 10g, Radix Et Rhizoma Notopterygii (*Qiang Huo*), 10g, Radix Et Rhizoma Rhei (*Da Huang*), 6g, Radix Rubrus Paeoniae Lactiflorae (*Chi Shao*), 10g, Radix Angelicae Sinensis (*Dang Gui*), 6g, Radix Ligustici Wallichii (*Chuan Xiong*), 10g, Radix Ledebouriellae Divaricatae (*Fang Feng*), 10g, Herba Equiseti Hiemalis (*Mu Zei*), 10g

3. Heat evils deep-lying in the network vessels

Symptoms: Slight reddening of the whites of the eyes with unevenly scattered fine vessels on the surface of the whites which are persistent, photophobia, tearing, slight itching and sore eyes which worsen in the afternoon

Therapeutic principles: Course heat and dispel stasis

Acupuncture & moxibustion:

Tai Yang (M-HN-9) *Zan Zhu* (Bl 2)	Together, these points unblock the network vessels in the eyes to free the flow of qi and blood.
Qu Chi (LI 11) *He Gu* (LI 4)	These are large intestine channel points which connect with the eyes indirectly and together course heat.
San Yin Jiao (Sp 6)	When used with *He Gu*, moves the qi and dispels stasis

Chinese medicinal formula: *Tui Re San* (Abate Heat Powder)

Ingredients: Radix Rubrus Paeoniae Lactiflorae (*Chi Shao*), 10g, Rhizoma Coptidis Chinensis (*Huang Lian*), 6g, Caulis Akebiae (*Mu*

Tong), 5g, Cortex Phellodendri (*Huang Bai*), 10g, Radix Scutellariae Baicalensis (*Huang Qin*), 10g, uncooked Radix Rehmanniae (*Sheng Di*), 10g, Fructus Gardeniae (Jasminoidis (*Zhi Zi*), 6g, Cortex Radicis Moutan (*Dan Pi*), 10g, Radix Angelicae Sinensis (*Dang Gui*), 6g, Radix Glycyrrhizae (*Gan Cao*), 3g

However, for minor cases manifesting sparsely scattered fine vessels on the surface of the whites of the eyes, discomfort and slight itching in the eyes, and slight tearing, one should use *Tui Chi San* (Abate Red Powder) in order to clear the lungs and move the blood.

Ingredients: Cortex Radicis Mori Albi (*Sang Bai Pi*), 10g, Radix Glycyrrhizae (*Gan Cao*), 10g, Radix Scutellariae Baicalensis (*Huang Qin*), 10g, Radix Platycodi Grandiflori (*Jie Geng*), 6g, Cortex Radicis Moutan (*Dan Pi*), 6g, Radix Trichosanthis Kirlowii (*Tian Hua Fen*), 10g, Radix Rubrus Paeoniae Lactiflorae (*Chi Shao*), 10g, Radix Angelicae Sinensis (*Dang Gui*), 10g, Semen Trichosanthis Kirlowii (*Gua Lou Ren*), 10g

4. Alcohol toxins brewing internally

Symptoms: Patients with this pattern have a history of alcohol addiction. In this pattern, the whites of the eyes gradually turn yellowish-red accompanied by dryness and itching. There may also be symptoms associated with damp heat brewing internally. Other symptoms include slimy, yellow tongue fur, and a soggy, rapid pulse.

Therapeutic principles: Clear heat and disinhibit dampness

Acupuncture & moxibustion:

Tong Zi Liao (GB 1)	Together, these points clear heat and resolve
Zan Zhu (Bl 1)	toxins when pricked to induce bleeding.
Yin Ling Quan (Sp 9)	Together, these points clear heat and disinhibit
San Yin Jiao (Sp 6)	dampness when needled with draining method.
Nei Ting (St 44)	

Chinese medicinal formula: Modified *Yin Chen Wu Ling San* (Artemisia Capillaris Five [Ingredients] Poria Powder)

Ingredients: Herba Artemisiae Capillaris (*Yin Chen Hao*), 10g, Rhizoma Alismatis (*Ze Xie*), 10g, Sclerotium Polypori Umbellati (*Zhu Ling*), 10g, Sclerotium Poriae Cocos (*Fu Ling*), 10g, Rhizoma Atractylodis Macrocephalae (*Bai Zhu*), 10g, Ramulus Cinnamomi Cassiae (*Gui Zhi*), 6g, Flos Puerariae (*Ge Hua*), 15g, Flos Dolichoris Lablab (*Bai Bian Hua*), 10g

5. Exuberant liver/gallbladder fire

Symptoms: Reddening of the whites of the eyes with burning pain, in some severe cases, red vessels scattered randomly on the surface of the whites, hot tearing, profuse eye discharge, distention of the eyes, aversion to heat, headache, especially at the vertex and in the temples, a bitter taste in the mouth, dry throat, lateral costal pain and distention, dark-colored urine, constipation, a red tongue, and a wiry, rapid pulse

Therapeutic principles: Clear and drain the liver and gallbladder

Acupuncture & moxibustion:

Feng Chi (GB 20)	Clears and drains fire in the gallbladder channel when needled with draining method
Tong Zi Liao (GB 1) *Zan Zhu* (Bl 2) *Shao Shang* (Lu 11)	Together, these points drain heat and dispel stasis when pricked to induce bleeding.
He Gu (LI 4)	Source point of the hand *yang ming* channel; clears heat in the head and eyes when needled with draining method
Xing Jian (Liv 2)	Spring point of the liver channel; drains liver fire when needled with draining method

Chinese medicinal formula: *Long Dan Xie Gan Tang* (Gentiana Drain the Liver Decoction)

Ingredients: Radix Gentianae Scabrae (*Long Dan Cao*), 6g, Rhizoma Alismatis (*Ze Xie*), 10g, Caulis Akebiae (*Mu Tong*), 5g, Semen Plantaginis (*Che Qian Zi*), 10g, Radix Angelicae Sinensis (*Dang Gui*), 6g, Radix Bupleuri (*Chai Hu*), 6g, uncooked Radix Rehmanniae (*Sheng Di*), 10g, Fructus Gardeniae Jasminoidis (*Zhi Zi*), 10g, Radix Scutellariae Baicalensis (*Huang Qin*), 10g, Radix Glycyrrhizae (*Gan Cao*), 3g

6. Yin vacuity of the liver & kidneys

Symptoms: Many of these patients are weak and have a history of chronic disease. The whites of the eyes look slightly red. The progression of the disease is slow. It attacks intermittently with several onsets per year. Other symptoms are low back and knee pain and weakness, vexatious heat in the five hearts, tidal fever, night sweats, and a fine, rapid pulse.

Therapeutic principles: Enrich water to moisten wood, clear the liver and drain fire

Acupuncture & moxibustion:

Zan Zhu (Bl 2)	Together, these points clear heat and dispel stasis
Tai Yang (M-HN-9)	when the needle is inserted in the direction of the eye and needled with draining method.
Tai Chong (Liv 3)	Clears the liver and drains fire when needled with draining method
Yong Quan (Ki 1)	Leads heat downward and drains fire when needled with draining method
Tai Xi (Ki 3)	Enriches water to moisten wood when needled with supplementing method

Chinese medicinal formula: *Shi Zhen Tang* (Ten Pearls Decoction)

Ingredients: Uncooked Radix Rehmanniae (*Sheng Di*), 10g, Radix Angelicae Sinensis (*Dang Gui*), 10g, Radix Albus Paeoniae Lactiflorae (*Bai Shao*), 10g, Cortex Radicis Lycii Chinensis (*Di Gu Pi*), 6g, Tuber Asparagi Cochinensis (*Tian Dong*), 6g, Rhizoma Anemarrhenae Asphodeloidis (*Zhi Mu*), 10g, Cortex Radicis Moutan (*Dan Pi*), 6g, Tuber Ophiopogonis Japonici (*Mai Dong*), 10g, Radix Panacis Ginseng (*Ren Shen*), 3g, Radix Glycyrrhizae (*Gan Cao*), 3g

12
Mydriasis *(Tong Shen San Da)*

This refers to dilatation of the pupils of the eyes. It is a serious symptom which calls for immediate care. Otherwise it may result in blindness.

Disease causes, disease mechanisms:

I. Dual vacuity of qi & yin

Dual vacuity of qi and yin may arise from exuberant fire of the heart and liver which consumes the qi and damages yin. It may also be due to febrile disease. Qi is responsible for astringing and, if there is qi vacuity, the pupil of the eyes may become dilated due to lack of this power of the qi to astringe the pupil. Moreover, the pupils' normal function depends on yin essence from the viscera. If there is yin vacuity, the pupils may not be sufficiently nourished and thus they may dilate.

2. Yin vacuity fire flaming upward

Yin vacuity may result from chronic disease, aging, sexual taxation, etc. Being vacuous, yin may fail to check yang. Therefore, yin vacuity fire comes into existence. If this fire then flames upward and attacks the eyes, the network vessels of the eyes may become disharmonious and the flow of qi, blood, and fluids there may become inhibited. Due to retention of fluids and blood, mydriasis may occur.

3. Phlegm fire blocking the portals

Spleen vacuity typically leads to accumulation of dampness which, with time, may transform into phlegm, while liver depression may cause qi stagnation and this stagnated qi may transform into fire. If this fire combines with phlegm, it may then go upward to attack the eyes along the liver channel drafting with it the phlegm. Phlegm fire then disturbs the portals and blocks the network vessels in the eyes. This blockage may then lead to retention of fluids and blood locally. The heat burns in the pupil and dilatation of the pupil may occur.

4. Exuberant liver fire

Emotional disturbance, such as anger and frustration, may give rise to exuberant liver fire. If this fire flames upward along the channel and attacks the eyes, the network vessels in the eyes may be damaged. As a result, the fluids and blood in the pupils will not flow freely and the pupils may become dilated.

5. Traumatic injury to the pupils

A direct or indirect blow on the pupils of the eyes may damage the network vessels of the pupils. Qi stagnation and blood stasis may thus bring about retention of the fluids and blood in the pupils. Therefore, dilatation of the pupils occurs.

Treatment based on pattern discrimination:

I. Dual vacuity of qi & yin

Symptoms: Dilatation of the pupils, clouded vision, dryness in the eyes, dizziness and vertigo, fatigue, lack of strength, vexation, reduced sleep, dry mouth and throat, a red tongue with yellow fur, and a soggy, fine pulse

Therapeutic principles: Boost the qi and nourish yin

Acupuncture and moxibustion:

Jing Ming (Bl 1)   Together, these points shrink the pupils and
Yi Ming (M-HN-13)   brighten the eyes.

Qi Hai Shu (Bl 24)   Together, these points supplement the qi.
Guan Yuan Shu (Bl 26)

Tai Xi (Ki 3)   Together, these points nourish yin.
San Yin Jiao (Sp 6)

Chinese medicinal formula: Modified *Zi Yin Di Huang Wan* (Enrich Yin
Rehmannia Pills)

Ingredients: Prepared Radix Rehmanniae (*Shu Di*), 12g, Radix
Dioscoreae Oppositae (*Shan Yao*), 12g, Fructus Corni Officinalis (*Shan
Zhu Yu*), 10g, Fructus Schisandrae Chinensis (*Wu Wei Zi*), 10g, Tuber
Ophiopogonis Japonici (*Mai Dong*), 10g, Radix Astragali Membranacei
(*Huang Qi*), 15g, Pericarpium Citri Reticulatae (*Chen Pi*), 10g, Radix
Angelicae Sinensis (*Dang Gui*), 10g, Flos Chrysanthemi Morifolii (*Ju
Hua*), 12g, Fructus Lycii Chinensis (*Gou Qi Zi*), 10g, Semen Astragali
Complanati (*Sha Yuan Zi*), 10g, Semen Cuscutae Chinensis (*Tu Si Zi*), 10g

2. Yin vacuity fire flaming upward

Symptoms: Dilatation of the pupils, blurred vision, red eyes, eye
discharge which binds the eyelids together, tinnitus, deafness, low back
and knee pain and weakness, seminal emission, a red tongue with
diminished fur, and a vacuous, fine, rapid pulse

Therapeutic principles: Enrich yin and downbear fire

Acupuncture & moxibustion:

Feng Chi (GB 20)   Together, these points downbear fire and
Tai Yang (M-HN-9)   harmonize the network vessels in the eyes to
Jing Ming (Bl 1)   move the fluids, qi, and blood.

Tai Xi (Ki 3)　　　　Together, these points nourish yin to downbear
San Yin Jiao (Sp 6)　fire.

Chinese medicinal formula: Modified *Xie Shen Tang* (Drain the Kidneys Decoction)

Ingredients: Fructus Lycii Chinensis (*Gou Qi Zi*), 18g, uncooked Radix Rehmanniae (*Sheng Di*), 10g, Cortex Phellodendri (*Huang Bai*), 10g, Rhizoma Anemarrhenae Asphodeloidis (*Zhi Mu*), 10g, Tuber Ophiopogonis Japonici (*Mai Dong*), 10g, Fructus Corni Officinalis (*Shan Zhu Yu*), 10g, Radix Albus Paeoniae Lactiflorae (*Bai Shao*), 6g, Radix Angelicae Sinensis (*Dang Gui*), 6g, Fructus Schisandrae Chinensis (*Wu Wei Zi*), 10g, Sclerotium Poriae Cocos (*Fu Ling*), 6g, Magnetitum (*Ci Shi*), 15g, Massa Medica Fermentata (*Shen Qu*), 6g, calcined Concha Margaritiferae (*Zhen Zhu Mu*), 15g

3. Phlegm fire blocking the portals

Symptoms: Dilatation of the pupils, blurred vision, distending pain in the eyeballs, forehead, and supraorbital bone, fever, thirst, vomiting with foamy vomitus, slimy tongue fur, and a wiry, glossy pulse

Therapeutic principles: Transform phlegm and clear heat

Acupuncture & moxibustion:

Feng Chi (GB 20)　　Together, these points unblock the network
Yu Yao (M-HN-6)　　vessels, move the qi and blood, and free the flow
Tai Yang (M-HN-9)　of the fluids.

Feng Long (St 40)　Together, these points transform phlegm to open
Nei Guan (Per 6)　　the portals of the eyes.

Da Zhui (CV 14)　　Together, these points clear heat and drain fire.
He Gu (LI 4)

Chinese medicinal formula: *Qing Tan Yin* (Clear Phlegm Drink)

Ingredients: Rhizoma Pinelliae Ternatae (*Ban Xia*), 10g, Pericarpium Citri Reticulatae (*Chen Pi*), 10g, Rhizoma Arisaematis (*Tian Nan Xing*), 10g, Radix Trichosanthis Kirlowii (*Tian Hua Fen*), 10g, Fructus Gardeniae Jasminoidis (*Zhi Zi*), 10g, Gypsum Fibrosum (*Shi Gao*), 15g, Radix Scutellariae Baicalensis (*Huang Qin*), 10g, Sclerotium Poriae Cocos (*Fu Ling*), 10g, Fructus Citri Aurantii (*Zhi Ke*), 6g, Pulvis Indigonis (*Qing Dai*), 5g

4. Exuberant liver fire

Symptoms: Dilatation of the pupils, painful distention of the eyes, dim vision, red eyes and facial complexion, chest oppression and pain in the lateral costal regions, vexation and agitation, belching, reduced food intake, a red tongue with thin fur, and a wiry pulse

Therapeutic principles: Regulate the liver, rectify the qi, and drain fire

Acupuncture & moxibustion:

Feng Chi (GB 20)	Drains liver fire and brightens the eyes
Jing Ming (Bl 1) *Yang Bai* (GB 14)	Together, these points harmonize the network vessels to promote the flow of the fluids.
Tai Chong (Liv 3) *Qi Men* (Liv 14)	Together, these points regulate the liver and rectify the qi.

Additions & subtractions: If there is constipation, add *Shang Ju Xu* (St 37).

Chinese medicinal formula: Modified *Tiao Qi Tang* (Regulate the Qi Decoction)

Ingredients: Rhizoma Cyperi Rotundi (*Xiang Fu*), 12g, Pericarpium Citri Reticulatae (*Chen Pi*), 10g, Radix Angelicae Sinensis (*Dang Gui*), 6g, Radix Albus Paeoniae Lactiflorae (*Bai Shao*), 12g, uncooked Radix Rehmanniae (*Sheng Di*), 6g, Rhizoma Coptidis Chinensis (*Huang Lian*), 6g, Rhizoma Anemarrhenae Asphodeloidis (*Zhi Mu*), 6g, Fructus Citri

Aurantii (*Zhi Ke*), 6g, Spica Prunellae Vulgaris (*Xia Ku Cao*), 10g, Semen Cassiae Torae (*Jue Ming Zi*), 10g

5. Traumatic injury to the pupils

Symptoms: Dilatation of the pupils, clouded vision, painful distention in the head and eyes or even bleeding into the pupil, painful swelling of the eyelid, a dull-colored tongue, and a wiry or choppy pulse

Therapeutic principles: Harmonize the constructive and transform stasis, enrich the kidneys and boost the essence

Acupuncture & moxibustion:

Jing Ming (Bl 1)	Together, these points unblock the network vessels in
Cheng Qi (St 1)	the eyes and move qi and blood.
Feng Chi (GB 20)	

Ge Shu (Bl 17)	Together, these points enrich the kidneys and boost
Gan Shu (Bl 18)	the essence at the same time as transforming stasis.
Shen Shu (Bl 23)	

Chinese medicinal formula: Modified *Da Huang Dang Gui San* (Rhubarb & Dang Gui Powder)

Ingredients: Radix Et Rhizoma Rhei (*Da Huang*), 6g, Radix Angelicae Sinensis (*Dang Gui*), 10g, Flos Carthami Tinctorii (*Hong Hua*), 10g, Lignum Sappan (*Su Mu*), 10g, Flos Chrysanthemi Morifolii (*Ju Hua*), 10g, Herba Equiseti Hiemalis (*Mu Zei*), 10g, Fructus Gardeniae Jasminoidis (*Zhi Zi*), 6g, prepared Radix Rehmanniae (*Shu Di*), 12g, Fructus Corni Officinalis (*Shan Zhu Yu*), 10g, Fructus Lycii Chinensis (*Gou Qi Zi*), 12g, Semen Cuscutae Chinensis (*Tu Si Zi*), 12g

13
Ciliary Hyperemia *(Chi Mai Chuan Jing)*

This refers to dilation of the blood vessels in the eyes. These dilated blood vessels start from either the inner or the outer canthus or both at the same time. They then travel laterally across the surface of the whites of the eyes. Usually, both eyes are involved.

Disease causes, disease mechanisms:

I. Replete fire in the heart channel

Replete fire may be the result of addiction to spicy food which leads to heat brewing in the spleen, or from emotional disturbance which transforms fire. If this heat or fire enters and brews in the heart channel, over time, this heat or fire will ascend along the heart channel and accumulate in the canthus. This is because the two canthi pertain to the heart according to five wheel doctrine. If heat accumulates in the blood vessels of the whites of the eyes, ciliary hyperemia will occur.

2. Vacuity fire in the heart channel

Taxation of the vision or overthinking may eventually consume heart yin. If heart yin becomes vacuous, vacuity fire may be engendered. If such vacuity fire flames upward along the heart channel and accumulates in the blood vessels of the canthi, ciliary hyperemia will occur.

3. Kidney essence depletion

Sexual intemperance is usually the cause of kidney essence depletion. In this disease, however, depletion mainly arises from replete fire and vacuity fire in the heart channel as described above in 1 and 2. If fire in the heart channel is not drained, not only will ciliary hyperemia linger, but the heart will absorb kidney yin from below and render kidney essence vacuous. In that case, evil qi is weak and so is the correct qi. Therefore, ciliary hyperemia lingers on and on.

Treatment based on pattern discrimination:

I. Replete fire in the heart channel

Symptoms: Thick, red, dilated blood vessels beginning from the canthus and running transversely through the whites of the eyes, itching, roughness, and a pricking sensation in the eyes, profuse eye discharge, headache, vexatious heat, dry mouth and throat, in some cases, sores on the tongue and in the mouth, constipation, dark, yellow urine, a red tongue tip with yellow fur, and a rapid, replete pulse

Therapeutic principles: Clear the heart and drain fire

Acupuncture & moxibustion:

Tai Yang (M-HN-9)   Together, these points drain fire when pricked to
Zan Zhu (Bl 2)   induce bleeding.

Feng Chi (GB 20)   Drains fire and brightens the eyes

Lao Gong (Per 8)   Drains heart fire

Additions & subtractions: If heart fire is persistent, choose two of the twelve spring points each time alternately and prick to bleed. If there are sores on the tongue and in the mouth, add *Si Feng* (M-UE-9).

Chinese medicinal formula: *Xie Xin Tang* (Drain the Heart Decoction) plus *Dao Chi San* (Abduct the Red Powder)

Ingredients: Rhizoma Coptidis Chinensis (*Huang Lian*), 6g, Radix Scutellariae Baicalensis (*Huang Qin*), 6g, Radix Et Rhizoma Rhei (*Da Huang*), 6g, uncooked Radix Rehmanniae (*Sheng Di*), 12g, Caulis Akebiae (*Mu Tong*), 5g, Herba Lophatheri Gracilis (*Dan Zhu Ye*), 6g, Radix Glycyrrhizae (*Gan Cao*), 3g

2. Vacuity fire in the heart channel

Symptoms: Slightly red, fine, and sparsely scattered blood vessels on the surface of the whites of the eyes, itching and discomfort in the eyes, vexation, insomnia, a red tongue with diminished fur, and a fine, rapid pulse

Therapeutic principles: Enrich yin and clear heat

Acupuncture & moxibustion:

Jing Ming (Bl 1) *Feng Chi* (GB 20)	Together, these point clear heat and move qi and blood.
Xin Shu (Bl 15) *Pi Shu* (Bl 20) *Shen Shu* (Bl 23)	Together, these points nourish heart and kidney yin.

Chinese medicinal formula: Modified *Zhi Bai Di Huang Wan* (Anemarrhena & Phellodendron Rehmannia Pills)

Ingredients: Uncooked Radix Rehmanniae (*Sheng Di*), 12g, Radix Dioscoreae Oppositae (*Shan Yao*), 6g, Fructus Corni Officinalis (*Shan Zhu Yu*), 6g, Cortex Radicis Moutan (*Dan Pi*), 10g, Semen Plantaginis (*Che Qian Zi*), 10g, Sclerotium Poriae Cocos (*Fu Ling*), 6g, Cortex Phellodendri (*Huang Bai*), 10g, Rhizoma Anemarrhenae Asphodeloidis (*Zhi Mu*), 9g, Tuber Ophiopogonis Japonici (*Mai Dong*), 10g

3. Kidney essence depletion

Symptoms: Fine, red blood vessels in and near the canthus, slight reddening of the whites of the eyes, dry eyes, blurred vision, tinnitus, deafness, low back and knee pain and weakness, seminal emission, premature ejaculation, night sweats, a red tongue with little fur, and a fine, forceless pulse

Therapeutic principles: Supplement the kidneys and replenish essence

Acupuncture & moxibustion:

Jing Ming (Bl 1) *Tai Yang* (M-HN-9)	Together, these points harmonize the network vessels and dispel evils.
Shen Shu (Bl 23) *Zhi Shi* (Bl 52)	Together, these points supplement the kidneys and replenish essence.

Chinese medicinal formula: Modified *Zuo Gui Wan* (Restore the Left [Kidney] Pills)

Ingredients: Prepared Radix Rehmanniae (*Shu Di*), 10g, Radix Dioscoreae Oppositae (*Shan Yao*), 10g, Fructus Corni Officinalis (*Shan Zhu Yu*), 10g, Fructus Lycii Chinensis (*Gou Qi Zi*), 12g, Semen Cuscutae Chinensis (*Tu Si Zi*), 12g, Fructus Ligustri Lucidi (*Nu Zhen Zi*), 12g, Gelatinum Cornu Cervi (*Lu Jiao Jiao*), 5g, Gelatinum Plastri Testudinis (*Gui Ban Jiao*), 5g, Fructus Mori Albi (*Sang Shen*), 10g

Remarks: Though effective, acupuncture can only work as an auxiliary therapy for ciliary hyperemia. It is, therefore, advisable to use Chinese internal medicine in combination with acupuncture.

14
Myopia *(Jin Shi)*

Myopia is more commonly called near-sightedness. It refers to the ability to clearly see nearby objects, while vision of distant objects is defective. Congenital myopia is not covered below.

Disease causes, disease mechanisms:

1. Heart yang vacuity

Heart yang vacuity mainly arises from internal damage and taxation or prolonged reading with improper posture or in dim light. Normal eyesight relies on spirit light (*shen guang*) which has its source in the life-gate fire while its ruler is the heart. Therefore, if heart yang becomes vacuous, this spirit light cannot be invigorated nor can it cast far afield. Hence myopia occurs.

2. Liver/kidney vacuity

Congenital insufficiency and sexual intemperance can lead to kidney vacuity. The wind wheel (*i.e.*, the cornea and iris) pertains to the liver, while the water wheel (*i.e.*, the pupil) belongs to the kidneys. These two wheels are crucial to the function of vision and their normal function depends on the nourishment of essence from the five viscera. "The kidneys receive and store the essence of the viscera and bowels" and "The liver opens into the portal of the eyes." Therefore, if there is liver/kidney vacuity, there may be myopia.

Treatment based on pattern discrimination:

I. Heart yang vacuity

Symptoms: Defective vision of distant objects. No other remarkable discomfort can be noticed except, in some cases, a drained white facial complexion, heart palpitations, lassitude of the spirit, a pale tongue, and a weak pulse.

Therapeutic principles: Supplement the heart and boost the qi, quiet the spirit and settle the will

Acupuncture & moxibustion:

Feng Chi (GB 20) *Tong Zi Liao* (GB 1) *Zan Zhu* (Bl 2) *Cheng Qi* (St 1) *Jing Ming* (Bl 1) *Si Zhu Kong* (TB 23) *Si Bai* (St 2) *Shou San Li* (LI 10) *He Gu* (LI 4)	Most of the yang channels meet in or around the eyes. Therefore, all the points selected can unblock the network vessels in the eyes, free the flow of qi and blood, and soothe the sinews of the eyes so as to sharpen the vision.
Shen Men (Ht 7) *Xin Shu* (Bl 15) *Nei Guan* (Per 6)	Together, these points supplement the heart, boost the qi, and quiet the spirit.

Note: The points in the first group should be used alternately, selecting 3-4 points each treatment in addition to the second group of points. The treatment should be done daily for 20 minutes each time. Twelve treatments equal 1 course of treatment. If the patient does not respond after 5 such courses, other therapies should be recommended.

Chinese medicinal formula: Modified *Ding Zhi Wan* (Stabilize the Will Pills)

Ingredients: Radix Panacis Ginseng (*Ren Shen*), 5g, Sclerotium Pararadicis Poriae Cocos (*Fu Shen*), 10g, Rhizoma Acori Graminei (*Shi Chang Pu*), 10g, Radix Polygalae Tenuifoliae (*Yuan Zhi*), 10g, Semen Astragali Complanati (*Sha Yuan Zi*), 10g, Semen Cuscutae Chinensis (*Tu Si Zi*), 10g, Fructus Rubi Chingii (*Fu Pen Zi*), 10g

2. Liver/kidney vacuity

Symptoms: Defective vision of distant objects, black, flowery (*i.e.*, blurred) vision follows gradually. Other symptoms may include dizziness, tinnitus, profuse dreaming, low back and knee pain and weakness, impotence, seminal emission, dribbling discharge of urine after voidings, a pale tongue, and a fine, weak pulse.

Therapeutic principles: Enrich and supplement the liver and kidneys, boost the essence, and brighten the eyes

Acupuncture & moxibustion: The treatment is the same as that for heart yang vacuity pattern. However, the points *Shen Men*, *Xin Shu*, and *Nei Guan* should be subtracted, while the points *Gan Shu* (Bl 18), *Shen Shu* (Bl 23), and *San Yin Jiao* (Sp 6) should be added in order to enrich and supplement the liver and kidneys.

Chinese medicinal formula: Modified *Bu Shen Ci Shi Wan* (Supplement the Kidneys Magnetite Pills)

Ingredients: Semen Cuscutae Chinensis (*Tu Si Zi*), 12g, Fructus Lycii Chinensis (*Gou Qi Zi*), 12g, Magnetitum (*Ci Shi*), 15g, Flos Chrysanthemi Morifolii (*Ju Hua*), 12g, Herba Cistanchis Deserticolae (*Rou Cong Rong*), 10g, Concha Haliotidis (*Shi Jue Ming*), 15g, prepared Radix Rehmanniae (*Shu Di*), 12g, Fructus Ligustri Lucidi (*Nu Zhen Zi*), 10g

Remarks: Acupuncture is effective, especially for juvenile pseudo-myopia. However, it is not indicated for congenital near-sightedness.

15
Far-sightedness *(Yuan Shi)*

Far-sightedness refers to the ability to see distant objects more clearly than those nearby.

Disease causes, disease mechanisms:

I. Yin essence vacuity

Yin essence vacuity arises from sexual intemperance, dietary irregularity, bodily taxation, or grief with tears. Visual acuity depends on sufficient nourishment by yin essence. Without sufficient nourishment, the portals of the eye cannot focus the spirit light and thus far-sightedness may occur.

2. Yin vacuity, fire effulgence

Chronic disease and sexual intemperance can lead to yin vacuity, effulgent fire. Thus it is said, "Far-sightedness is due to fire and lack of water."

3. Dual vacuity of qi & blood

Dual vacuity of qi and blood may result from congenital insufficiency, a vacuous spleen and stomach, etc. Visual acuity relies upon the qi which invigorates the spirit light and on the blood which nourishes the eyes and focuses the spirit light. If there is dual vacuity of the qi and the blood, far-sightedness may thus occur.

4. Dual vacuity of yin & yang

This pattern is often encountered in elderly patients. Dual vacuity of yin and yang may arise from aging, chronic disease, and overtaxation in general or sexual taxation in particular. Yin is responsible for nourishing the eyes and focusing the spirit light, while yang is responsible for invigorating the spirit light and casting the spirit light far afield. Thus, if there is dual vacuity of yin and yang, myopia and far-sightedness may coexist. In the elderly, yin vacuity is often more severe than yang vacuity. Therefore, far-sightedness is often more severe than near-sightedness in the aged.

Treatment based on pattern discrimination:

I. Yin essence vacuity

Symptoms: Inability to see near objects clearly, aching in the eyeballs on enduring looking, dizziness, tinnitus, low back and knee pain and weakness, dry mouth and throat; in some severe cases, seminal emission, night sweats, loosening of the teeth, a red tongue with diminished fur, and a fine, rapid pulse

Therapeutic principles: Enrich the kidneys and boost the essence

Acupuncture & moxibustion:

Zan Zhu (Bl 2) *Tai Yang* (M-HN-9)	Together, these points clear and disinhibit the head and eyes.
Zeng Guang	An empirical point for visual problems which is located halfway between *Zan Zhu* [Bl 2] and *Yu Yao* [M-HN-6].
Gan Shu (Bl 18) *Shen Shu* (Bl 23)	Together, these points enrich the kidneys and boost essence.

Additions & subtractions: If there is headache, painful distention in the eyes, or aching in the eyeballs, add *Feng Chi* (GB 20) and *Yin Tang* (M-HN-3). For this purpose, puncture *Yin Tang* with the tip of the needle directed toward the eyes.

Chinese medicinal formula: Modified *Liu Wei Di Huang Wan* (Six Flavors Rehmannia Pills)

Ingredients: Prepared Radix Rehmanniae (*Shu Di*), 12g, Fructus Corni Officinalis (*Shan Zhu Yu*), 10g, Radix Dioscoreae Oppositae (*Shan Yao*), 10g, Cortex Radicis Moutan (*Dan Pi*), 6g, Semen Plantaginis (*Che Qian Zi*), 6g, Sclerotium Poriae Cocos (*Fu Ling*), 6g, Fructus Lycii Chinensis (*Gou Qi Zi*), 12g, Semen Cuscutae Chinensis (*Tu Si Zi*), 10g, Fructus Ligustri Lucidi (*Nu Zhen Zi*), 10g

2. Yin vacuity, fire effulgence

Symptoms: Inability to see near objects clearly and persistently, slight reddening of the canthus, dizziness, tinnitus, low back and knee pain and weakness, tidal fever, flushed cheeks, night sweats, a crimson tongue, and a fine, wiry, rapid pulse

Therapeutic principles: Enrich yin and downbear fire

Acupuncture & moxibustion:

Feng Chi (GB 20)	Together, these points clear and disinhibit the
Zan Zhu (Bl 2)	head and eyes.
Tai Yang (M-HN-9)	

Guang Ming (GB 37)	Together, these points enrich yin, downbear fire,
Tai Xi (Ki 3)	and brighten the eyes.
San Yin Jiao (Sp 6)	

Chinese medicinal formula: Modified *Zhi Bai Di Huang Wan*

(Anemarrhena & Phellodendron Rehmannia Pills)

Ingredients: Prepared Radix Rehmanniae (*Shu Di*), 12g, Fructus Corni Officinalis (*Shan Zhu Yu*), 10g, Radix Dioscoreae Oppositae (*Shan Yao*), 10g, Cortex Radicis Moutan (*Dan Pi*), 6g, Semen Plantaginis (*Che Qian Zi*), 6g, Sclerotium Poriae Cocos (*Fu Ling*), 6g, Fructus Lycii Chinensis (*Gou Qi Zi*), 12g, Semen Cuscutae Chinensis (*Tu Si Zi*), 10g, Fructus Ligustri Lucidi (*Nu Zhen Zi*), 10g, Cortex Phellodendri (*Huang Bai*), 10g, Rhizoma Anemarrhenae Asphodeloidis (*Zhi Mu*), 12g

3. Dual vacuity of the qi & blood

Symptoms: Inability to see near objects clearly, aching in the eyes on enduring looking (in some cases, this aching may refer to the orbit and the forehead), a dull facial complexion, heart palpitations or racing of the heart, dizziness, insomnia, shortness of breath, lassitude of the spirit, loss of appetite, a pale tongue with diminished fur, and a fine, forceless pulse

Therapeutic principles: Supplement and boost the qi and blood

Acupuncture & moxibustion:

Bai Hui (GV 20)   Upbears the qi and blood to nourish the eyes

Zan Zhu (Bl 2)   Together, these points help brighten the eyes.
Zeng Guang (see above p. 86)

Zu San Li (St 36)   Together, these points fortify the spleen to
Pi Shu (Bl 20)   promote the engendering and transformation of qi
Wei Shu (Bl 19)   and blood.

Chinese medicinal formula: Modified *Ba Zhen Tang* (Eight Pearls Decoction)

Ingredients: Prepared Radix Rehmanniae (*Shu Di*), 12g, Radix

Angelicae Sinensis (*Dang Gui*), 10g, Radix Albus Paeoniae Lactiflorae (*Bai Shao*), 10g, Radix Ligustici Wallichii (*Chuan Xiong*), 6g, Radix Codonopsis Pilosulae (*Dang Shen*), 10g, Rhizoma Atractylodis Macrocephalae (*Bai Zhu*), 10g, Sclerotium Poriae Cocos (*Fu Ling*), 10g, mix-fried Radix Glycyrrhizae (*Zhi Gan Cao*), 6g, Semen Cuscutae Chinensis (*Tu Si Zi*), 12g, Fructus Lycii Chinensis (*Gou Qi Zi*), 12g

4. Dual vacuity of yin & yang

Symptoms: Reduced visual acuity but better ability to see distant than near objects, a cold body and chilled limbs, a pale tongue with white fur, and a deep, fine pulse

Therapeutic principles: Support yang and boost yin

Acupuncture & moxibustion:

Zeng Guang (see above) *Yi Ming* (M-HN-13)	Empirical points for brightening the eyes
Gan Shu (Bl 18) *Shen Shu* (Bl 23)	Together, these points boost yin.
Pi Shu (Bl 20)	Engenders qi and blood
Ming Men (GV 4)	Supports yang

Note: Moxibustion can be applied to the points on the back.

Chinese medicinal formula: Modified *You Gui Wan* (Restore the Right [Kidney] Pills)

Ingredients: Semen Cuscutae Chinensis (*Tu Si Zi*), 12g, Cortex Cinnamomi Cassiae (*Rou Gui*), 3g, Gelatinum Cornu Cervi (*Lu Jiao Jiao*), 5g, Radix Dioscoreae Oppositae (*Shan Yao*), 10g, prepared Radix Rehmanniae (*Shu Di*), 12g, Fructus Corni Officinalis (*Shan Zhu Yu*),

10g, Fructus Lycii Chinensis (*Gou Qi Zi*), 12g, Radix Angelicae Sinensis (*Dang Gui*), 6g, Semen Astragali Complanati (*Sha Yuan Zi*), 10g, Fructus Rubi Chingii (*Fu Pen Zi*), 10g, Fructus Ligustri Lucidi (*Nu Zhen Zi*), 10g

Remarks: Acupuncture therapy can relieve the discomfort of the eyes and can also improve the eyesight to some extent. However, far-sightedness from dual vacuity of yin and yang does not respond well to acupuncture therapy alone.

16
Decreased Visual Acuity *(Shi Li Jian Tui)*

Hypopsia or decreased visual acuity refers to reduced ability to see objects clearly.

Disease causes, disease mechanisms:

I. Turbid evils harassing above

Dietary irregularity is the main cause in this case which can lead to damp heat brewing internally and phlegm dampness which, with time, may transform into heat. If damp heat or phlegm heat fumes and steams, this will affect the flow of fluids and qi and blood in the eyes. Thus, visual acuity may be reduced.

2. Qi stagnation & blood stasis

Emotional disturbance may lead to liver depression and cause qi stagnation and blood stasis. This may then transform into fire. Because "The liver opens into the portals of the eyes," qi stagnation and blood stasis due, in turn, to liver depression may eventually affect the eyes. If the fire transformed from qi stagnation goes upward to the eyes along the liver channel, it will brew in the eyes in combination with stagnated qi and blood stasis, possibly causing reduced visual acuity.

3. Insufficiency of the liver & kidneys

Insufficiency of the liver and kidneys may arise from aging, sexual taxation, constitutional vacuity, and chronic disease. In Chinese medicine there are the sayings: "The kidneys receive and store the essence from all the viscera and bowels," "The eyes can see only when the liver receives sufficient blood," and "The liver stores blood." Thus, if there is insufficiency of the liver and kidneys, the eyes may be deprived of sufficient nourishment and visual acuity may consequently be reduced.

4. Dual vacuity of the heart & spleen

Dual vacuity of the heart and spleen may result from chronic disease, taxation, or postpartum. If there is dual vacuity of the heart blood and spleen qi, the blood will be insufficient and the eyes will not be properly nourished. Therefore, the visual acuity may be reduced.

Treatment based on pattern discrimination:

I. Turbid evils harassing above

Symptoms: Indistinct vision, in some cases, accompanied by black, flowery vision, tinted vision, or seeing large things as small. Other symptoms may include heavy-headedness, chest oppression, reduced food intake, a bitter taste in the mouth, yellow, scant urine, slimy, yellow tongue fur, and a soggy, rapid pulse. When phlegm is predominant, there is abdominal fullness, profuse phlegm, a bitter taste and sliminess in the mouth, slimy, yellow tongue fur, and a slippery, rapid pulse.

Therapeutic principles: Disinhibit dampness and clear heat, eliminate phlegm and transform turbidity

Acupuncture & moxibustion:

Jing Ming (Bl 1)   Together, these points clear heat and free the
Feng Chi (GB 20)   flow of qi and blood.
Zeng Guang (see above p. 86)

He Gu (LI 4)   Together, these points move the qi and fortify the
San Yin Jiao (Sp 6)   spleen, eliminate phlegm and transform turbidity.

Chinese medicinal formulas:

If the pattern is damp heat: Modified *San Ren Tang* (Three Seed Decoction)

Ingredients: Talcum (*Hua Shi*), 10g, Medulla Tetrapanacis Papyriferi (*Tong Cao*), 6g, Cortex Magnoliae Officinalis (*Hou Po*), 10g, Semen Pruni Armeniacae (*Xing Ren*), 6g, Fructus Cardamomi (*Bai Dou Kou*), 10g, Semen Coicis Lachryma-jobi (*Yi Yi Ren*), 20g, Herba Lophatheri Gracilis (*Dan Zhu Ye*), 10g, Rhizoma Pinelliae (*Ban Xia*), 10g, Semen Plantaginis (*Che Qian Zi*), 10g, Semen Leonuri Heterophylli (*Chong Wei Zi*), 12g, Fructus Gardeniae Jasminoidis (*Zhi Zi*), 10g

If the pattern is phlegm heat: Modified *Wen Dan Tang* (Warm the Gallbladder Decoction)

Ingredients: Resina Olibani (*Ru Xiang*), 10g, Rhizoma Pinelliae Ternatae (*Ban Xia*), 10g, Pericarpium Citri Reticulatae (*Chen Pi*), 10g, Fructus Immaturi Citri Aurantii (*Zhi Shi*), 6g, Sclerotium Poriae Cocos (*Fu Ling*), 10g, bile-processed Rhizoma Arisaematis (*Dan Nan Xing*), 6g, Semen Plantaginis (*Che Qian Zi*), 10g, Semen Leonuri Heterophylli (*Chong Wei Zi*), 12g, Rhizoma Coptidis Chinensis (*Huang Lian*), 6g

2. Qi stagnation & blood stasis

Symptoms: Vague pain in the eyeballs, reduced visual acuity, in some cases, a tinted shade in the middle of the visual field, or visual distortion of objects. Other symptoms may include inhibited emotions, dizziness, pain in the lateral costal region, a bitter taste in the mouth, a dry throat, and a wiry, fine, rapid pulse.

Therapeutic principles: Clear heat and soothe the liver, move the qi and quicken the blood

Acupuncture & moxibustion:

Tong Zi Liao (GB 1) *Zuan Zhu* (Bl 2)	Together, these points quicken the blood and eliminate stasis when pricked to induce bleeding.
Guang Ming (GB 37) *Tai Chong* (Liv 3)	Together, these points soothe the liver and brighten the eyes.
He Gu (LI 4) *San Yin* Jiao (Sp 6)	Together, these points move the qi and quicken the blood to eliminate stasis.

Chinese medicinal formula: Modified *Dan Zhi Xiao Yao San* (Moutan & Gardenia Rambling Powder)

Ingredients: Radix Angelicae Sinensis (*Dang Gui*), 10g, Radix Albus Paeoniae Lactiflorae (*Bai Shao*), 10g, Rhizoma Atractylodis Macrocephalae (*Bai Zhu*), 6g, Radix Bupleuri (*Chai Hu*), 6g, Sclerotium Poriae Cocos (*Fu Ling*), 6g, mix-fried Radix Glycyrrhizae (*Zhi Gan Cao*), 3g, Herba Menthae Haplocalycis (*Bo He*), 3g, Cortex Radicis Moutan (*Dan Pi*), 10g, Fructus Gardeniae Jasminoidis (*Zhi Zi*), 6g, Radix Salviae Miltiorrhizae (*Dan Shen*), 10g, Radix Ligustici Wallichii (*Chuan Xiong*), 10g, Semen Leonuri Heterophylli (*Chong Wei Zi*), 15g

3. Insufficiency of the liver & kidneys

Symptoms: Dry eyes, indistinct vision or visual distortion of objects, dizziness, tinnitus, dream-disturbed sleep, low back and knee pain and weakness, a red tongue, and a fine pulse

Therapeutic principles: Supplement and boost the liver and kidneys

Acupuncture & moxibustion:

Zeng Guang (see above) *Qiu Hou* (M-HN-8)	Together, these points brighten the eyes.

Gan Shu (Bl 18)	Together, these points supplement and boost the liver and kidneys.
Pi Shu (Bl 20)	
Shen Shu (Bl 23)	

Chinese medicinal formula: Modified *Qi Ju Di Huang Wan* (Lycium & Chrysanthemum Rehmannia Pills)

Ingredients: Prepared Radix Rehmanniae (*Shu Di*), 12g, Fructus Corni Officinalis (*Shan Zhu Yu*), 10g, Radix Dioscoreae Oppositae (*Shan Yao*), 10g, Semen Plantaginis (*Che Qian Zi*), 10g, Cortex Radicis Moutan (*Dan Pi*), 6g, Sclerotium Poriae Cocos (*Fu Ling*), 6g, Fructus Lycii Chinensis (*Gou Qi Zi*), 12g, Flos Chrysanthemi Morifolii (*Ju Hua*), 12g, Fructus Ligustri Lucidi (*Nu Zhen Zi*), 10g

4. Dual vacuity of the heart & spleen

Symptoms: Dry eyes, indistinct vision or visual distortion of objects, a lusterless facial complexion, dizziness, heart palpitations, reduced food intake, lassitude of the spirit, a pale tongue, and a fine pulse

Therapeutic principles: Nourish the heart and boost the spleen, supplement and quicken the blood

Acupuncture & moxibustion:

Zeng Guang (see above)	Together, these points free the flow of qi and blood and brighten the eyes.
Feng Chi (GB 20)	
Yang Lao (SI 6)	

Xin Shu (Bl 15)	Together, these points nourish the heart and boost the spleen, supplement and quicken the blood.
Pi Shu (Bl 20)	
Ge Shu (Bl 17)	
Gan Shu (Bl 18)	

Chinese medicinal formula: Modified *Ren Shen Yang Rong Tang* (Ginseng Nourish the Constructive Decoction)

Ingredients: Radix Astragali Membranacei (*Huang Qi*), 12g, Radix Panacis Ginseng (*Ren Shen*), 6g, Sclerotium Poriae Cocos (*Fu Ling*), 10g, Rhizoma Atractylodis Macrocephalae (*Bai Zhu*), 10g, mix-fried Radix Glycyrrhizae (*Zhi Gan Cao*), 6g, Radix Angelicae Sinensis (*Dang Gui*), 10g, Radix Albus Paeoniae Lactiflorae (*Bai Shao*), 10g, Cortex Cinnamomi Cassiae (*Rou Gui*), 3g, Fructus Schisandrae Chinensis (*Wu Wei Zi*), 10g, Radix Polygalae Tenuifoliae (*Yuan Zhi*), 6g, Pericarpium Citri Reticulatae (*Chen Pi*), 6g, Radix Ligustici Wallichii (*Chuan Xiong*), 10g, Radix Salviae Miltiorrhizae (*Dan Shen*), 10g

17
Night Blindness *(Ye Mang)*

Night blindness refers to normal vision during the daytime with reduced visual acuity in faint light or at night. It is mainly encountered in young people and women.

Disease causes, disease mechanisms:

I. Insufficiency of liver blood

Insufficiency of liver blood may arise due to congenital vacuity or great loss of blood. Based on the sayings, "The liver opens into the portals of the eyes" and "The eyes can see only when the liver receives sufficient blood," if liver blood becomes vacuous, the eyes may not receive enough nourishment. Thus the spirit light may become weak, leading to the occurrence of night blindness.

2. Liver/kidney yin vacuity

Liver/kidney yin vacuity may be due to insufficiency of liver blood, constitutional yin vacuity, aging, chronic disease, or sexual intemperance. "The eyes can see only when liver receives sufficient blood," "The essence from all the viscera and bowels pours into the eyes," and "The kidney, governing water, receives and stores essence from all the viscera and bowels." Thus, if there is liver/kidney yin vacuity, the eyes may be deprived of sufficient nourishment and the spirit light will be affected. Therefore, when the light is dim, the visual capacity may be reduced.

3. Spleen qi vacuity

Spleen qi vacuity may result from dietary irregularity, taxation, and overthinking. When spleen qi is vacuous and center qi is insufficient, clear yang cannot be upborne. In that case, the eyes will not receive enough nourishment and the visual capacity may be reduced. Thus there may be night blindness.

4. Spleen/kidney yang vacuity

Spleen/kidney yang vacuity is mainly the result of enduring spleen qi vacuity, constitutional yang vacuity, enduring disease, and aging. If spleen yang is vacuous, first, clear yang cannot be upborne in order to nourish the eyes. Secondly, engendering and transformation will be affected. Thus there will be less qi and blood engendered and transformed to nourish the eyes. This is made worse by the fact that kidney yang vacuity may lead to exuberant yin. Such exuberant yin, in turn, may obstruct the network vessels in the eyes and hence lead to qi and blood stagnation and stasis in the region of the eyes. This may then affect the visual acuity resulting in night blindness.

5. Dual vacuity of the qi & blood

Dual vacuity of the qi and blood may develop from chronic disease which consumes the qi and blood and constitutional spleen vacuity which results in insufficiency in engendering and transforming the qi and blood. If there is qi vacuity, blood cannot be warmed and moved to nourish the eyes. If there is blood vacuity, the spirit light will not be enriched. Therefore, the visual capacity may reduced and night blindness may occur.

Treatment based on pattern discrimination:

I. Insufficiency of liver blood

Symptoms: Indistinct vision or inability to see objects clearly after sunset, dry, itchy eyes, photophobia, frequent blinking, in some severe cases, ulcers and eye screen on the dark of the eyes. Other symptoms may include dizziness, heart palpitations, a pale tongue with thin fur, and a fine, wiry pulse.

Therapeutic principles: Nourish the liver and supplement the blood

Acupuncture & moxibustion:

Jing Ming (Bl 1)	All of these are points for eye diseases which
Zan Zhu (Bl 2)	unblock the network vessels and free the flow of qi
Si Bai (St 2)	and blood in the local region. Select 3-4 of these
Feng Chi (GB 20)	points alternately each treatment.
Tong Zi Liao (GB 1)	
Zeng Guang (see above)	
Guang Ming (GB 37)	

Additions & subtractions: Add *Gan Shu* (Bl 18) and *Pi Shu* (Bl 20) if there is insufficiency of liver blood. Add *Gan Shu* (Bl 18), *Shen Shu* (Bl 23), and *Tai Xi* (Ki 3) if there is liver/kidney yin vacuity. Add *Zu San Li* (St 36) and *San Yin Jiao* (Sp 6) if there is spleen qi vacuity. Add *Pi Shu* (Bl 20), *Shen Shu* (Bl 23), *Guan Yuan Shu* (Bl 26), and *Qi Hai Shu* (Bl 24) if there is spleen/kidney yang vacuity. Add *Qi Hai* (CV 6), *Pi Shu* (Bl 20), and *Ge Shu* (Bl 17) if there is dual vacuity of the qi and blood.

Chinese medicinal formula: Modified *Zhuan Guang Wan* (Return Light Pills)

Ingredients: Uncooked Radix Rehmanniae (*Sheng Di*), 10g, prepared Radix Rehmanniae (*Shu Di*), 10g, Sclerotium Poriae Cocos (*Fu Ling*),

10g, Radix Ligustici Wallichii (*Chuan Xiong*), 10g, Fructus Viticis (*Man Jing Zi*), 10g, Radix Dioscoreae Oppositae (*Shan Yao*), 6g, Flos Chrysanthemi Morifolii (*Ju Hua*), 12g, Radix Angelicae Sinensis (*Dang Gui*), 10g, Fructus Mori Albi (*Sang Shen*), 10g, Fructus Lycii Chinensis (*Gou Qi Zi*), 10g, Excrementum Vespertilionis Murini (*Ye Ming Sha*), 2g, powdered

Remarks: Patients with this pattern of night blindness should include beef, pig, lamb, or chicken livers in their diet.

2. Liver/kidney yin vacuity

Symptoms: Normal vision during the daytime but reduced visual acuity with a narrow visual field at night, dryness and discomfort in the eyes, vexation, reduced sleep, low back and knee pain and weakness, dizziness, tinnitus, dry mouth, seminal emission, a red tongue with little fur, and a fine, rapid pulse

Therapeutic principles: Enrich and supplement the liver and kidneys, nourish the heart and quiet the spirit

Acupuncture & moxibustion: See the prescription for insufficiency of liver blood above.

Chinese medicinal formula: Modified *Qi Ju Di Huang Wan* (Lycium & Chrysanthemum Rehmannia Pills)

Ingredients: Prepared Radix Rehmanniae (*Shu Di*), 12g, Fructus Corni Officinalis (*Shan Zhu Yu*), 10g, Radix Dioscoreae Oppositae (*Shan Yao*), 6g, Cortex Radicis Moutan (*Dan Pi*), 6g, Semen Plantaginis (*Che Qian Zi*), 10g, Sclerotium Poriae Cocos (*Fu Ling*), 6g, Rhizoma Atractylodis (*Cang Zhu*), 10g, Excrementum Vespertilionis Murini (*Ye Ming Sha*), 2g, powdered, Fructus Lycii Chinensis (*Gou Qi Zi*), 12g, Flos Chrysanthemi Morifolii (*Ju Hua*), 12g

Additions & subtractions: Add Radix Salviae Miltiorrhizae (*Dan Shen*), 10g, Radix Cyathulae (*Chuan Niu Xi*), 10g, and Radix Ilicis Pubescentis (*Mao Dong Qing*), 10g, to quicken blood and transform stasis if there is a turbid color in the retina. If vacuity heat is strong, add Rhizoma Anemarrhenae Asphodeloidis (*Zhi Mu*), 10g, and Cortex Phellodendri (*Huang Bai*), 10g.

3. Spleen qi vacuity

Symptoms: Inability to see objects clearly after dusk falls, a narrow visual field, a white facial complexion, lassitude of the spirit, reduced food intake, lack of strength, a pale tongue with thin, white fur, and a fine, weak pulse

Therapeutic principles: Supplement the spleen and boost the qi

Acupuncture & moxibustion: See the prescription for insufficiency of liver blood above.

Chinese medicinal formula: Modified *Bu Zhong Yi Qi Tang* (Supplement the Center & Boost the Qi Decoction)

Ingredients: Radix Astragali Membranacei (*Huang Qi*), 15g, Radix Codonopsis Pilosulae (*Dang Shen*), 10g, Rhizoma Atractylodis (*Cang Zhu*), 10g, Radix Angelicae Sinensis (*Dang Gui*), 6g, Pericarpium Citri Reticulatae (*Chen Pi*), 6g, Rhizoma Cimicifugae (*Sheng Ma*), 3g, Radix Bupleuri (*Chai Hu*), 3g, Excrementum Vespertilionis Murini (*Ye Ming Sha*), 2g, powdered, Radix Ligustici Wallichii (*Chuan Xiong*), 10g, Radix Salviae Miltiorrhizae (*Dan Shen*), 10g

4. Spleen/kidney yang vacuity

Symptoms: Inability to see objects at night, loss of visual acuity, a narrow visual field, cold body and chilled limbs, low back and knee pain and weakness, impotence, premature ejaculation, fifth-watch, (*i.e.*, cockcrow), diarrhea, long voidings of clear urine, in some cases, dribbling after urinary voiding, a fat, pale tongue with slimy, white fur, and a deep, fine pulse but faint at the cubit position

Therapeutic principles: Warm and supplement the spleen and kidneys

Acupuncture & moxibustion: See the prescription for insufficiency of liver blood above.

Chinese medicinal formula: Modified *You Gui Wan* (Restore the Right [Kidney] Pills)

Ingredients: Prepared Radix Rehmanniae (*Shu Di*), 12g, Radix Dioscoreae Oppositae (*Shan Yao*), 10g, Fructus Corni Officinalis (*Shan Zhu Yu*), 10g, Semen Cuscutae Chinensis (*Tu Si Zi*), 12g, Fructus Lycii Chinensis (*Gou Qi Zi*), 12g, Cortex Eucommiae Ulmoidis (*Du Zhong*), 10g, Radix Lateralis Praeparatus Aconiti Carmichaeli (*Fu Zi*), 3g, Cortex Cinnamomi Cassiae (*Rou Gui*), 3g, Radix Angelicae Sinensis (*Dang Gui*), 6g, Gelatinum Cornu Cervi (*Lu Jiao Jiao*), 5g, Radix Ligustici Wallichii (*Chuan Xiong*), 10g, Radix Cyathulae (*Chuan Niu Xi*), 10g

5. Dual vacuity of the qi & blood

Symptoms: Inability to see objects after dusk, a narrow visual field, a drained white facial complexion, heart palpitations, insomnia, lassitude of the spirit, lack of strength, shortness of breath, spontaneous perspiration, a pale tongue, and a fine, weak pulse

Therapeutic principles: Supplement and boost the qi and blood

Acupuncture & moxibustion: See the prescription for insufficiency of liver blood above.

Chinese medicinal formula: Modified *Chai Hu Shen Zhu Tang* (Bupleurum, Ginseng & Atractylodes Decoction)

Ingredients: Radix Bupleuri (*Chai Hu*), 3g, Radix Panacis Ginseng (*Ren Shen*), 6g, Rhizoma Atractylodis Macrocephalae (*Bai Zhu*), 12g, prepared Radix Rehmanniae (*Shu Di*), 10g, Radix Albus Paeoniae Lactiflorae (*Bai Shao*), 10g, Radix Ligustici Wallichii (*Chuan Xiong*), 10g, Radix Angelicae Sinensis (*Dang Gui*), 10g, Pericarpium Citri Reticulatae Viride (*Qing Pi*), 3g, mix-fried Radix Glycyrrhizae *(Zhi Gan Cao)*, 3g, Excrementum Vespertilionis Murini (*Ye Ming Sha*), 2g, powdered, Fructus Lycii Chinensis (*Gou Qi Zi*), 12g

18
Sudden Blindness *(Bao Ming)*

Sudden blindness refers to a sudden, rapid loss of visual acuity which may, in fact, be total. This may occur in one or both eyes.

Disease causes, disease mechanisms:

Normal visual capacity depends on the warming and nourishing functions of the qi and blood. Any factors leading to an abrupt disturbance of the qi and blood supply may give rise to sudden blinding.

I. Heat entering the constructive & blood aspects

This is mainly seen in the final stage of febrile diseases when warm heat evils fall inward into the constructive and blood aspects. This results in the reckless moving of blood due to blood heat. If this reckless blood dashes upward to the head and eyes, damaging the ligation of the eyes, sudden blindness may occur.

2. Phlegm heat congesting above

Phlegm heat may be engendered from addiction to smoking, alcohol, or sweet, fatty and spicy foods. If phlegm heat brews internally and then goes upward to congest in the clear portals, the network vessels in the eyes may become blocked. If the clear yang becomes blocked, it then cannot be upborne to warm and nourish the eyes. Thus sudden blindness may occur.

3. Exuberant liver fire

Liver fire exuberance may be due to emotional disturbance, such as anger and depression. Depression may transform into fire, while anger can trigger the ascension of liver fire. "The liver opens into the portals of the eyes" and the liver channel connects with the ligation of the eyes. If liver fire flames upward along the channel and suddenly damages the network vessels in the eyes, sudden blinding may occur.

4. Liver wind stirring internally

Sexual intemperance, aging, or chronic disease may lead to yin vacuity of the liver and kidneys. Liver yang is checked by liver/kidney yin. If there is yin vacuity of the liver and kidneys, liver yang typically will become hyperactive and may, if severe, transform into wind. If this wind drafts upward suddenly causing the disorderly flow of qi and blood, the network vessels may become blocked abruptly and thus the eyes may be suddenly deprived of their nourishment. Hence, sudden blinding may occur.

5. Yin vacuity, fire effulgence

Yin vacuity, fire effulgence may be due to constitutional yin vacuity, overthinking which consumes heart yin surreptitiously, or febrile diseases which damage yin. If water fails to check fire, fire will tend to flame upward. If up-flaming yin vacuity fire damages or suddenly blocks the network vessels in the eyes, leading to an abrupt shortage of qi and blood supplied to the eyes, sudden blinding may result.

6. Qi & blood stasis and blockage

Emotional depression can lead to liver depression and qi stagnation which may and typically does give rise to blood stasis over time. If stasis causes a sudden blockage in the network vessels in the eyes, sudden blinding may occur.

Treatment based on pattern discrimination:

I. Heat entering the constructive & blood aspects

Symptoms: Sudden blindness, high fever, thirst, clouded spirit, delirious speech, maculopapular eruptions in some cases, a crimson red tongue with completely peeled tongue fur, and a fine, rapid pulse

Therapeutic principles: Clear the constructive and resolve toxins, cool the blood and stop bleeding

Acupuncture & moxibustion:

Jing Ming (Bl 1)	These are key points for eye diseases. They
Tong Zi Liao (GB 2)	brighten the eyes. *Tong Zi Liao* is pricked to bleed.

Guan Chong (TB 1)	Together, these points clear heat, cool the blood,
Zhong Chong (Per 9)	and stop bleeding when pricked to bleed.
Nei Ying Xiang (M-HN-35)	

Chinese medicinal formulas:

For evils in the constructive aspect: *Qing Ying Tang* (Clear the Constructive Decoction)

Ingredients: Cornu Bubali (*Shui Niu Jiao*), 30g, uncooked Radix Rehmanniae (*Sheng Di*), 15g, Radix Scrophulariae Ningpoensiss (*Xuan Shen*), 15g, Folium Bambusae (*Zhu Ye*), 10g, Rhizoma Coptidis Chinensis (*Huang Lian*), 10g, Tuber Ophiopogonis Japonici (*Mai Dong*), 10g, Radix Salviae Miltiorrhizae (*Dan Shen*), 10g, Flos Lonicerae Japonicae (*Yin Hua*), 10g, Fructus Forsythiae Suspensae (*Lian Qiao*), 10g

For evils in the blood aspect: Modified *Xi Jiao Di Huang Tang* (Rhinoceros Horn & Rehmannia Decoction)

Ingredients: Cornu Bubali (*Shui Niu Jiao*), 30g, uncooked Radix Rehmanniae (*Sheng Di*), 15g, Radix Rubrus Paeoniae Lactiflorae (*Chi Shao*), 12g, Cortex Radicis Moutan (Dan *Pi),* 12g

If evils enter the pericardium: *An Gong Niu Huang Wan* (Quiet the Palace Bezoar Pills)

Ingredients: Calculus Bovis (*Niu Huang*), 0.5g, not decocted, Tuber Curcumae (*Yu Jin*), 10g, Cornu Bubali (*Shui Niu Jiao*), 30g, Rhizoma Coptidis Chinensis (*Huang Lian*), 10g, Cinnabar (*Zhu Sha*), 0.5g, not decocted, Borneol (*Bing Pian*), 0.5g, not decocted, Secretio Moschi Moschiferi (*She Xiang*), 0.05g, not decocted, Margarita (*Zhen Zhu*), 0.5g, powdered, Fructus Gardeniae Jasminoidis (*Zhi Zi*), 10g, Realgar (*Xiong Huang*), 0.5g, not decocted, Radix Scutellariae Baicalensis (*Huang Qin*), 10g

Decoct the *Yu Jin, Shui Niu Jiao, Huang Lian, Huang Qin,* and *Zhi Zi* first. Then take the other ingredients washed down with the warm decoction. The dosage is for one day.

2. Phlegm heat congesting above

Symptoms: Rapid reduction in visual acuity or even total blindness, vertigo, heavy-headedness, chest oppression, vexation and agitation, reduced food intake, nausea, thick phlegm, a bitter taste in the mouth, slimy, yellow tongue fur, and a wiry, slippery pulse

Therapeutic principles: Flush the phlegm and open the portals

Acupuncture & moxibustion:

Jing Ming (Bl 1)   Together, these points unblock the network
Qiu Hou (M-HN-8)   vessels and open the portals.

Feng Chi (GB 20)	A gallbladder point which is good for eye diseases; brightens the eyes
Tian Zhu (Bl 10)	A bladder point which is good for eye diseases; helps *Jing Ming* free the flow of the qi and blood
Feng Long (St 40)	The network point of the stomach and a key point for transforming the phlegm
Nei Ting (St 44)	The spring point of the stomach and a key point for clearing replete heat. Together, these points clear heat and flush phlegm.

Chinese medicinal formula: Modified *Di Tan Tang* (Flush Phlegm Decoction)

Ingredients: Rhizoma Pinelliae Ternatae (*Ban Xia*), 10g, bile-processed Rhizoma Arisaematis (*Dan Nan Xing*), 6g, Pericarpium Citri Reticulatae (*Chen Pi*), 10g, Fructus Immaturus Citri Aurantii (*Zhi Shi*), 10g, Sclerotium Poriae Cocos (*Fu Ling*), 10g, Rhizoma Acori Graminei (*Shi Chang Pu*), 10g, Caulis Bambusae In Taeniis (*Zhu Ru*), 10g, Bombyx Batryticatus (*Jiang Can*), 10g, Lumbricus (*Di Long*), 3g, powdered, Radix Ligustici Wallichii (*Chuan Xiong*), 10g, Radix Cyathulae (*Chuan Niu Xi*), 10g

Additions & subtractions: If heat is severe, add Rhizoma Coptidis Chinensis (*Huang Lian*), 6g, and Radix Scutellariae Baicalensis (*Huang Qin*), 10g.

3. Exuberant liver fire

Symptoms: Rapid reduction in visual acuity or even total blindness which may occur in one or both eyes, pain or pressure in the eyeballs, headache, tinnitus, a bitter taste in the mouth, dry throat, a red face and eyes, vexation and agitation, pain in the lateral costal region, a red tongue with yellow fur, and a wiry, rapid pulse

Therapeutic principles: Clear the liver and drain fire

Acupuncture & moxibustion:

Jing Ming (Bl 1) *Tong Zi Liao* (GB 2)	Together, these points unblock the network vessels and open the portals.
Xia Xi (GB 43) *Xing Jian* (Liv 2)	"Spring points course heat." Therefore, the combination of these two spring points strongly drains liver fire when needled with draining method.

Additions & subtractions: If the eyes are distended, add *Guan Chong* (TB 1) and prick to induce bleeding. If there is pain and distention in the lateral costal region, add *Yang Ling Quan* (GB 34) and *Qi Men* (Liv 14).

Chinese medicinal formula: Modified *Long Dan Xie Gan Tang* (Gentiana Drain the Liver Decoction)

Ingredients: Radix Gentianae Scabrae (*Long Dan Cao*), 6g, Rhizoma Alismatis (*Ze Xie*), 6g, Caulis Akebiae (*Mu Tong*), 5g, Semen Plantaginis (*Che Qian Zi*), 12g, Radix Bupleuri (*Chai Hu*), 6g, uncooked Radix Rehmanniae (*Sheng Di*), 10g, Radix Scutellariae Baicalensis (*Huang Qin*), 10g, Fructus Gardeniae Jasminoidis (*Zhi Zi*), 10g, Cortex Radicis Moutan (*Dan Pi*),10g, Radix Ilicis Pubescentis (*Mao Dong Qing*), 10g, Radix Rubrus Paeoniae Lactiflorae (*Chi Shao*), 10g

4. Liver wind stirring internally

Symptoms: The onset of blindness often comes suddenly after a violent bout of anger. Other symptoms may include dizziness, tinnitus, occasional tidal flushing of the face, vexation and agitation, irascibility, a bitter taste in the mouth, a red tongue with yellow fur, and a wiry pulse. In some cases, there is also low back and knee pain and weakness, seminal emission, lassitude of the spirit, a crimson tongue, and a fine pulse.

Therapeutic principles: Calm the liver and subdue yang, enrich yin and extinguish the wind

Acupuncture & moxibustion:

Jing Ming (Bl 1) *Tong Zi Liao* (GB 2)	Together, these points unblock the network vessels and open the portals.
Tai Chong (Liv 3)	Calms the liver and subdues yang
Yong Quan (Ki 1)	Leads blood downward to prevent wind stroke
Tai Xi (Ki 3) *San Yin Jiao* (Sp 6)	Together, these points enrich yin to check yang and extinguish the wind.

Chinese medicinal formula: Modified *Tian Ma Gou Teng Yin* (Gastrodia & Uncaria Drink)

Ingredients: Rhizoma Gastrodiae Elatae (*Tian Ma*), 10g, Ramulus Uncariae Cum Uncis (*Gou Teng*), 15g, Concha Haliotidis (*Shi Jue Ming*), 15g, Fructus Gardeniae Jasminoidis (*Zhi Zi*), 10g, Radix Scutellariae Baicalensis (*Huang Qin*), 6g, Cortex Eucommiae Ulmoidis (*Du Zhong*), 6g, Radix Achyranthis Bidentatae (*Huai Niu Xi*), 6g, Semen Leonuri Heterophylli (*Chong Wei Zi*), 10g, Ramulus Loranthi Seu Visci (*Sang Ji Sheng*), 10g, Sclerotium Pararadicis Poriae Cocos (*Fu Shen*), 10g, Caulis Polygoni Multiflori (*Ye Jiao Teng*), 10g, Flos Chrysanthemi Morifolii (*Ju Hua*), 15g, Semen Cassiae Torae (*Cao Jue Ming*), 10g

5. Yin vacuity, fire effulgence

Symptoms: Dizziness and vertigo, blindness often preceded by a vision of smoke ascending and scattering slowly which later turns to a sheet of red light. Other symptoms may include tidal fever with red cheeks, heart palpitations, night sweats, vexatious heat of the five hearts, a red tongue with scant fur, and a fine, forceless pulse.

Therapeutic principles: Enrich yin and downbear fire

Acupuncture & moxibustion:

Feng Chi (GB 20)	Together, these points course the liver and brighten
Tian Zhu (Bl 10)	the eyes.

Tai Chong (Liv 3)	The source point of the liver; downbears the fire with draining method.
Fu Liu (Ki 7)	The river point of the kidney channel.
Tai Xi (Ki 3)	The source point of the kidney channel
	Together, these points enhance the action of enriching yin to subdue yang

Additions & subtractions: If there are night sweats, add *Xin Shu* (Bl 15) and *Shen Shu* (Bl 23).

Chinese medicinal formula: Modified *Zhi Bai Di Huang Wan* (Anemarrhena & Phellodendron Rehmannia Pills)

Ingredients: Prepared Radix Rehmanniae (*Shu Di*), 12g, Fructus Corni Officinalis (*Shan Zhu Yu*), 10g, Radix Dioscoreae Oppositae (*Shan Yao*), 10g, Cortex Radicis Moutan (*Dan Pi*), 6g, Semen Plantaginis (*Che Qian Zi*), 12g, Sclerotium Poriae Cocos (*Fu Ling*), 10g, Rhizoma Anemarrhenae Asphodeloidis (*Zhi Mu*), 10g, Cortex Phellodendri (*Huang Bai*), 10g, Fructus Lycii Chinensis (*Gou Qi Zi*), 10g, Fructus Ligustri Lucidi (*Nu Zhen Zi*), 10g

6. Qi & blood stasis and blockage

Symptoms: Sudden blindness in one eye, depressed essence spirit, painful distention in the chest and lateral costal regions, fullness in the stomach and scant food intake, white tongue fur, and a wiry pulse. In severe cases, headache, a bitter taste in the mouth, and a fine, choppy pulse.

Therapeutic principles: In minor cases, course the liver and resolve depression, move the qi and quicken the blood. In severe cases, quicken the blood and transform stasis, move the qi and unblock the portals.

Acupuncture & moxibustion:

Jing Ming (Bl 1)	Together, these points move the qi, quicken the
Qiu Hou (M-HN-35)	blood, and unblock the network vessels and portals.
Feng Chi (GB 20)	Together, these points course the liver and
Guang Ming (GB 37)	brighten the eyes.
Ge Shu (Bl 17)	The meeting point of the blood; moves the qi, quickens the blood, and transforms stasis

Additions & subtractions: If there is a bitter taste in the mouth, add *Yang Ling Guan* (GB 34). For painful distention in the lateral costal regions, add *Qi Men* (Liv 14) and *Tai Chong* (Liv 3).

Chinese medicinal formula: Modified *Tong Qiao Huo Xue Tang* (Free the Portals & Quicken the Blood Decoction)

Ingredients: Radix Rubrus Paeoniae Lactiflorae (*Chi Shao*), 10g, Radix Ligustici Wallichii (*Chuan Xiong*), 10g, Semen Pruni Persicae (*Tao Ren*), 10g, Flos Carthami Tinctorii (*Hong Hua*), 10g, Radix Bupleuri (*Chai Hu*), 6g, Rhizoma Cyperi Rotundi (*Xiang Fu*), 6g, Fructus Tribuli Terrestris (*Bai Ji Li*), 10g, Spica Prunellae Vulgaris (*Xia Ku Cao*), 10g, Concha Haliotidis (*Shi Jue Ming*), 20g, Tuber Curcumae (*Yu Jin*), 10g, Radix Angelicae Sinensis (*Dang Gui*), 10g

Additions & subtractions: If there is bleeding in the eye ground, add Radix Pseudoginseng (*San Qi*), 3g, powdered, Pollen Typhae (*Pu Huang*), 10g, and Radix Rubiae Cordifoliae (*Qian Cao*), 10g.

19
Tinnitus & Deafness *(Er Ming & Er Long)*

Tinnitus is a subjective symptom in which the patient hears a ringing, roaring, hissing, or other such sound in their ears. Deafness refers to decreased auditory acuity to the point that daily life is affected, or the complete inability to perceive sounds.

Tinnitus and deafness may occur either independently or often simultaneously. In any case, they share the same disease causes and disease mechanisms. Moreover, in Chinese medicine, deafness is considered a severe form of tinnitus, while tinnitus is seen as a minor form of deafness. Therefore, they are dealt with here as one pathocondition.

Disease causes, disease mechanisms:

The ears are located in the cephalic part of the body, being one of the clear portals. It is said in Chinese medicine, "The ears are the gathering place of the vessels." Thus the ears have a close relationship with the other parts of the body and especially with the kidneys, liver, heart, gallbladder, spleen, and the sea of marrow. In addition, the capacity to hear relies on the nourishment of essence supplied by all the viscera and bowels by way of the channels and network vessels. Therefore, any factors which disturb this supply of nourishment or harass the clear portals may result in tinnitus and/or deafness.

1. Wind heat invading the lungs

Wind heat may be due to either directly contracted external wind heat, or externally contracted wind cold which has transformed into heat.

Commonly, external evils invading the body first attack the lungs. The lungs link with the ears via the network vessels. If wind heat in the lungs goes upward, first, this may lead to tinnitus if these evils harass the clear portals. Secondly, it may cause deafness if these evils create blockage in the network vessels of the ears and interrupt the supply of nourishment.

2. Exuberant liver fire

Exuberant liver fire may arise directly from strong anger which leads to excessive upbearing and effusing by the liver. It may also arise from depression which transforms fire. The liver channel has an exterior/interior relationship with the gallbladder channel. The gallbladder channel enters the ears from along its pathway behind the ears. If exuberant liver fire attacks above, tinnitus will occur when liver fire harasses the clear portals, and deafness will happen when this fire congests in or damages the network vessels of the ears.

3. Ascendant liver yang

Ascendant liver yang may be the result of the yin vacuity of the liver and kidneys. If yin cannot properly check liver yang, the later will ascend. As a result, the clear portals may be harassed by this ascendant liver yang and tinnitus and/or deafness may result.

4. Insufficiency of liver blood

Insufficiency of liver blood may be due to insufficiency of engendering and transforming by the spleen, great loss of blood, or chronic disease which consumes yin blood. The capacity to hear relies on the nourishment of essence and blood and "The liver stores the blood." Therefore, if there is liver blood insufficiency, the ears may not be sufficiently nourished. Thus tinnitus and/or deafness may occur.

5. Kidney yin vacuity

Kidney yin vacuity mainly comes from sexual intemperance, congenital insufficiency, aging, or chronic disease. It is said in Chinese medicine, "The kidneys open into the ears" and "The kidneys receive essence from all the viscera and bowels." If there is kidney yin vacuity, the ears may not be properly nourished. Therefore, tinnitus and/or deafness may occur.

6. Insufficiency of kidney qi

Insufficiency of kidney qi may result from aging, early or intemperate sexual activities, etc. If there is insufficiency of kidney qi, first, less kidney essence will be engendered and transformed since kidney qi and kidney essence mutually engender and transform into each other. Secondly, the kidneys will fail in their storage function, leading to essence loss and thus rendering kidney essence vacuous. "The kidneys open into the portals of the ears" and thus the capacity to hear relies on the nourishment mainly from kidney essence. Kidney qi engenders kidney essence, and essence engenders the marrow. The brain is the sea of marrow. If there is kidney qi vacuity, less marrow will be engendered. As a result, the marrow may not be able to fill up the cavity of the skull and may be shaken easily. "Shaking of the brain leads to tinnitus." Therefore, tinnitus may occur.

7. Breakdown of the interaction between the heart & kidneys

Breakdown of the interaction between the heart and kidneys may be the result of exuberant heart fire caused, in turn, by excess of the five emotions or from kidney yin vacuity caused by sexual intemperance, masturbation, etc. Physically, heart fire above should descend to interact with kidney water below and vice versa. If this fails to happen, either due to fire in the heart or yin vacuity of the kidneys, the interaction between the heart and kidneys may be broken. In that case, there may be heart fire flaming upward alone or invasion of the heart by ministerial fire whose lower source is the life-gate fire. In this latter case, ministerial fire combines with heart fire to flame upward. "The hand *shao yin* communicates with the ears through the network vessels." If heart fire flames upward and disturbs the clear portals, tinnitus and/or deafness may thus occur.

8. Spleen/stomach vacuity

Spleen/stomach vacuity may arise from constitutional insufficiency, dietary irregularity which damages the spleen and stomach, overtaxation, chronic disease, or overthinking, anxiety, and worry. The spleen is the source of engendering and transformation of the qi and blood. The capacity to hear relies on the warming and nourishment by the qi and blood. Therefore, if the spleen is vacuous, the ears may be deprived of sufficient nourishment. Hence, tinnitus and/or deafness may occur. In addition, when the spleen is vacuous, spleen qi is often rendered vacuous. In that case, the clear qi cannot be upborne to nourish the ears, and dampness cannot be transformed. This then may create blockage in the network vessels in the ears. Damp evils are a type of liquid and their nature is to flow. When it collects and blocks, deafness may occur. When it flows slowly, tinnitus may occur.

9. Phlegm fire

Phlegm fire can arise from dietary irregularity which damages the spleen, causing phlegm accumulation, or from emotional disturbance, resulting in liver depression/qi stagnation which may transform into fire. The foot *yang ming* channel directly connects with the ears. If fire goes upward with phlegm along the channel, tinnitus may occur if phlegm fire disturbs the clear portals, while deafness will occur if phlegm fire blocks the network vessels of the ears. In addition, phlegm evils are a type of liquid and their nature is to flow. If phlegm collects in and blocks the ear, deafness will happen. If it flows, tinnitus will occur.

10. Qi stagnation & blood stasis

Qi stagnation and blood stasis may be due to frustration which causes liver depression/qi stagnation or from trauma which leads to qi stagnation and blood stasis. Qi stagnation can result in blood stasis and vice versa. When there are qi stagnation and blood stasis, the ears cannot receive proper nourishment. As a result, tinnitus and/or deafness may occur.

Treatment based on pattern discrimination:

I. Wind heat invading the lungs

Symptoms: The onset is rapid and is often preceded by a common cold. There is a stifling distention in the ears. In some cases, the patient feels a blockage in the ears. Auditory acuity may be reduced in one or both the ears. The tinnitus sounds like the roaring of wind. Concomitant symptoms typically include nasal congestion, profuse nasal mucous, headache, fever, a red tongue with thin fur, and a floating, rapid pulse.

Therapeutic principles: Course and dissipate wind heat

Acupuncture & moxibustion:

Yi Feng (TB 17) *Ting Gong* (SI 19)	Together, these points course and dissipate wind heat in the ear and unblock the network vessels locally.
Si Du (TB 9)	A point on the triple burner which frees the flow of the channel qi to help *Yi Feng* open the portals and helps *He Gu* and *Pian Li* course and dissipate wind heat
He Gu (LI 4) *Pian Li* (LI 6)	Together, these points are a combination of source and network points which course the wind, dissipate the heat, and resolve the exterior.

Additions & subtractions: If there is fever, add *Da Zhui* (GV 14).

Chinese medicinal formula: Modified *Yin Qiao San* (Lonicera & Forsythia Powder)

Ingredients: Flos Lonicerae Japonicae (*Yin Hua*), 12g, Fructus Forsythiae Suspensae (*Lian Qiao*), 10g, Herba Menthae Haplocalycis (*Bo He*), 6g, Semen Praeparatus Sojae (*Dan Dou Chi*), 6g, Radix Platycodi Grandiflori (*Jie Geng*), 6g, Herba Schizonepetae Tenuifoliae (*Jing Jie*), 10g, Rhizoma Phragmitis Communis (*Lu Gen*), 10g, Folium Bambusae (*Zhu Ye*), 10g, Fructus Arctii Lappae (*Niu Bang Zi*), 10g, Radix Puerariae (*Ge Gen*), 15g, Rhizoma Acori Graminei (*Shi Chang Pu*), 10g, Radix Glycyrrhizae (*Gan Cao*), 3g

2. Exuberant liver fire

Symptoms: The tinnitus sounds like the roaring of a tide or thundering of a big bell. The deafness can be better and worse at intervals and is typically precipitated by anger. Other symptoms may include painful distention in the ears, ear blockage, headache, dizziness, a red face and eyes, a bitter taste in the mouth, dry throat, restless sleep, vexation and agitation, pain in the lateral costal regions, constipation, dark-colored urine, a red tongue with yellow fur, and a wiry, rapid, forceful pulse.

Therapeutic principles: Clear the liver and drain fire, open depression and unblock the portals

Acupuncture & moxibustion:

Yi Feng (TB 17)	These are *shao yang* channel points and the *shao*
Ting Hui (GB 2)	*yang* goes around the ear. They harmonize the network vessels in the ear and free the flow of qi and blood locally.

Zhong Zhu (TB 3)	These are important points of the triple burner,
Xia Xi (GB 43)	gallbladder, and liver which, when used in
Tai Chong (Liv 3)	combination, can strongly open depression and drain liver fire.

Additions & subtractions: Add *Zhi Gou* (TB 6) for constipation.

Chinese medicinal formula: Modified *Long Dan Xie Gan Tang* (Gentiana Drain the Liver Decoction)

Ingredients: Radix Gentianae Scabrae (*Long Dan Cao*), 6g, Rhizoma Alismatis (*Ze Xie*), 6g, Caulis Akebiae (*Mu Tong*), 5g, Semen Plantaginis (*Che Qian Zi*), 6g, Radix Bupleuri (*Chai Hu*), 6g, uncooked Radix Rehmanniae (*Sheng Di*), 10g, Radix Scutellariae Baicalensis (*Huang Qin*), 10g, Fructus Gardeniae Jasminoidis (*Zhi Zi*), 10g, Cortex Radicis Moutan (*Dan Pi*), 10g, Rhizoma Acori Graminei (*Shi Chang Pu*), 10g, Tuber Curcumae (*Yu Jin*), 10g

3. Ascendant liver yang

Symptoms: Tinnitus and/or deafness, dizziness, painful distention in the ears, a red face and eyes, insomnia, dry mouth and throat, low back and knee pain and weakness, a red tongue with scant liquids, and a wiry, fine, rapid pulse

Therapeutic principles: Enrich yin and subdue yang

Acupuncture & moxibustion:

Yi Feng (TB 17)   Together, these points unblock the network vessels
Ting Hui (GB 2)   and free the flow of the qi and blood in the ear.

Tai Chong (Liv 3)   Levels the liver and subdues yang

Tai Xi (Ki 3)   Together, these points enrich yin and subdue yang.
San Yin Jiao (Sp 6)

Chinese medicinal formula: Modified *Tian Ma Gou Teng Yin* (Gastrodia & Uncaria Decoction)

Ingredients: Rhizoma Gastrodiae Elatae (*Tian Ma*), 10g, Ramulus Uncariae Cum Uncis (*Gou Teng*), 15g, Concha Haliotidis (*Shi Jue*

Ming), 15g, Fructus Gardeniae Jasminoidis (*Zhi Zi*), 10g, Radix Scutellariae Baicalensis (*Huang Qin*), 10g, Cortex Eucommiae Ulmoidis (*Du Zhong*), 10g, Radix Achyranthis Bidentatae (*Huai Niu Xi*), 10g, Ramulus Loranthi Seu Visci (*Sang Ji Sheng*), 10g, Sclerotium Pararadicis Poriae Cocos (*Fu Shen*), 6g, Caulis Polygoni Multiflori (*Ye Jiao Teng*), 15g, Magnetitum (*Ci Shi*), 15g, Rhizoma Acori Graminei (*Shi Chang Pu*), 10g

4. Insufficiency of liver blood

Symptoms: Ringing in the ears like cicadas, better or worse at intervals, worse on taxation and in the afternoon, possible decreased auditory acuity, dizziness, a white, lusterless facial complexion, lusterless nails, dream-disturbed sleep, dry eyes, blurred vision, a pale tongue, and a fine pulse

Therapeutic principles: Enrich and supplement liver blood

Acupuncture & moxibustion:

Yi Feng (TB 17)	Together, these points unblock the network
Ting Hui (GB 2)	vessels and free the flow of the qi and blood in the ear.
San Yin Jiao (Sp 6)	Together, these points fortify the spleen to
Zu San Li (St 36)	engender the blood.
Ge Shu (Bl 17)	
to *Pi Shu* (Bl 21)	These points may be used alternatively in place of *San Yin Jiao* and *Zu San Li*. In which case, tap the points with a plum blossom needle.

Chinese medicinal formula: Modified *Si Wu Tang* (Four Ingredients Decoction)

Ingredients: Prepared Radix Rehmanniae (*Shu Di*), 12g, Radix Angelicae Sinensis (*Dang Gui*), 10g, Radix Albus Paeoniae Lactiflorae (*Bai Shao*), 10g, Radix Ligustici Wallichii (*Chuan Xiong*), 6g, Radix Bupleuri (*Chai Hu*), 3g, Rhizoma Acori Graminei (*Shi Chang Pu*), 10g, Fructus Mori Albi (*Sang Shen*), 10g

5. Kidney yin vacuity

Symptoms: Typically, a prolonged disease course, a low ringing in the ears like that of cicadas, deafness which gets worse gradually, dizziness, vertigo, insomnia, seminal emission, a dry mouth and throat, dimming of the vision, vexatious heat in the five hearts, night sweats, low back and knee aching and pain, a red tongue with thin fur, and a fine, rapid pulse

Therapeutic principles: Enrich and supplement kidney yin

Acupuncture & moxibustion:

Er Men (TB 21)	Together, these points harmonize the network
Ting Hui (GB 2)	vessels and unblock the portals.
Tai Xi (Ki 3)	The key yin points on the kidney channel;
Fu Liu (Ki 7)	together, they strongly enrich and supplement kidney yin to downbear fire.
San Yin Jiao (Sp 6)	Enriches yin to help downbear fire

Additions & subtractions: If there are night sweats, add *Yin Xi* (Ht 6).

Chinese medicinal formula: Modified *Er Long Zuo Ci Wan* (Deafness Left [Kidney] Good Pills)

Ingredients: Prepared Radix Rehmanniae (*Shu Di*), 12g, Radix Dioscoreae Oppositae (*Shan Yao*), 10g, Fructus Corni Officinalis (*Shan Zhu Yu*), 10g, Cortex Radicis Moutan (*Dan Pi*), 6g, Rhizoma Alismatis

(*Ze Xie*), 6g, Sclerotium Poriae Cocos (*Fu Ling*), 6g, Radix Bupleuri (*Chai Hu*), 3g, Magnetitum (*Ci Shi*), 15g, Rhizoma Acori Graminei (*Shi Chang Pu*), 10g

6. Insufficiency of kidney qi

Symptoms: Lingering tinnitus and/or deafness, ringing like that of cicadas which is worse at night, fear of cold, chilled limbs, low back and knee pain and weakness, seminal emission, impotence, long voiding of clear urine, fatigue, lack of strength, diminished food intake, loose stools, a drained white facial complexion, white tongue fur, and a fine, weak pulse

Therapeutic principles: Warm and supplement the kidney qi

Acupuncture & moxibustion:

Yi Feng (TB 17)	Together, these points upbear yang to warm and
Ting Hui (GB 2)	unblock the portals.
Bai Hui (GV 20)	

Guan Yuan (CV 4)	Together, when moxaed, these points warm and
Qi Hai (CV 6)	supplement the kidney qi.

Chinese medicinal formula: Modified *Cong Rong Wan* (Cistanches Pills)

Ingredients: Herba Cistanchis Deserticolae (*Rou Cong Rong*), 10g, Fructus Corni Officinalis (*Shan Zhu Yu*), 10g, Rhizoma Acori Graminei (*Shi Chang Pu*), 10g, Semen Cuscutae Chinensis (*Tu Si Zi*), 10g, Magnetitum (*Ci Shi*), 15g, Cortex Eucommiae Ulmoidis (*Du Zhong*), 10g, Rhizoma Drynariae (*Gu Sui Bu*), 10g, Cornu Parvum Cervi (*Lu Rong*), 1g, powdered

7. Breakdown of the interaction between the heart & kidneys

Symptoms: Tinnitus and reduced hearing capacity which are lingering and develop gradually, ringing in the ears which is not very loud and which is worse when there has been poor sleep, deafness more serious than tinnitus, vacuity vexation, insomnia, heart palpitations, amnesia, low back and knee pain and weakness, tidal fever, night sweats, short voiding of dark-colored urine, a red tongue with scant fur, and a fine, rapid pulse

Therapeutic principles: Enrich yin and downbear fire, communicate the heart and kidneys

Acupuncture & moxibustion:

Yi Feng (TB 17)	Together, these points harmonize the network
Ting Gong (SI 19)	vessels in the ear and unblock the portals.

Da Ling (Per 7)	Drains heart fire
Tai Xi (Ki 3)	Nourishes kidney yin
Yin Jiao (CV 7)	Communicates yin and yang
	Together, these points enrich yin and downbear fire in order to communicate the heart and kidneys.

Additions & subtractions: If there are night sweats, add *Yin Xi* (Ht 6) and *Fu Liu* (Ki 7).

Chinese medicinal formula: Modified *Huang Lian E Jiao Tang* (Coptis & Donkey Skin Glue Decoction)

Ingredients: Rhizoma Coptidis Chinensis (*Huang Lian*), 6g, Gelatinum Corii Asini (*E Jiao*), 5g, Radix Albus Paeoniae Lactiflorae (*Bai Shao*), 6g, Radix Scutellariae Baicalensis (*Huang Qin*), 6g, egg yolk, 1 piece, Magnetitum (*Ci Shi*), 20g, Rhizoma Acori Graminei (*Shi Chang Pu*), 10g

8. Spleen/stomach vacuity

Symptoms: Tinnitus and deafness which are worsened with taxation or standing up after squatting, a sudden, occasional empty, cold sensation in the ears, fatigue, lack of strength, scant food intake, abdominal distention after eating, a sallow yellow facial complexion, loose stools, pale lips and tongue, thin, white tongue fur, and a vacuous, weak pulse

Therapeutic principles: Supplement the center and boost the qi

Acupuncture & moxibustion:

Yi Feng (TB 17) *Ting Hui* (GB 2)	Together, these points harmonize the network vessels in the ear and unblock the portals.
Zu San Li (St 36) *Wei Shu* (Bl 21) *Pi Shu* (Bl 20)	Together, these points fortify the spleen to engender and transform qi and blood.

Chinese medicinal formula: Modified *Bu Zhong Yi Qi Tang* (Supplement the Center & Boost the Qi Decoction)

Ingredients: Radix Astragali Membranacei (*Huang Qi*), 15g, Radix Codonopsis Pilosulae (*Dang Shen*), 10g, Rhizoma Atractylodis Macrocephalae (*Bai Zhu*), 10g, Radix Angelicae Sinensis (*Dang Gui*), 6g, Pericarpium Citri Reticulatae (*Chen Pi*), 6g, Rhizoma Cimicifugae (*Sheng Ma*), 3g, Radix Bupleuri (*Chai Hu*), 3g, Rhizoma Acori Graminei (*Shi Chang Pu*), 10g, Radix Puerariae (*Ge Gen*), 10g, mix-fried Radix Glycyrrhizae (*Zhi Gan Cao*), 3g

9. Phlegm fire

Symptoms: Ringing which sounds like a tide and decreased auditory acuity, stifling blockage in the ears, a clouded head and heavy-headedness, fullness and oppression in the chest and stomach, cough with profuse phlegm, inhibited urination and defecation, a red tongue with slimy, yellow fur, and a wiry, slippery pulse

Therapeutic principles: Clear fire and transform phlegm, harmonize the stomach and downbear turbidity

Acupuncture & moxibustion:

Yi Feng (TB 17)	Together, these points unblock the network
Ting Hui (GB 2)	vessels and the portals.
Zhong Zhu (TB 3)	Together, these points free the flow of the triple
Nei Ting (St 44)	burner channel qi and drain heat.
Feng Long (St 40)	With *Nei Ting*, this poing transforms phlegm and
	drains phlegm fire.

Chinese medicinal formula: *Huang Lian Wen Dan Tang* (Coptis Warm the Gallbladder Decoction)

Ingredients: Caulis Bambusae In Taeniis (*Zhu Ru*), 6g, Rhizoma Pinelliae Ternatae (*Ban Xia*), 10g, Fructus Immaturus Citri Aurantii (*Zhi Shi*), 6g, Sclerotium Poriae Cocos (*Fu Ling*), 10g, Pericarpium Citri Reticulatae (*Chen Pi*), 10g, Rhizoma Coptidis Chinensis (*Huang Lian*), 6g, Radix Glycyrrhizae (*Gan Cao*), 3g

10. Qi stagnation & blood stasis

Symptoms: Sudden onset of tinnitus and/or deafness, dizziness, headache, vexation and agitation, distention and fullness in the chest and lateral costal regions, a dull, stagnant-looking tongue with thin fur, and a wiry, choppy pulse

Therapeutic principles: Move the qi, quicken the blood, and transform stasis

Acupuncture & moxibustion:

Yin Feng (TB 17) *Ting Hui* (GB 2)	Together, these points quicken the blood and unblock the network vessels in the ear.
He Gu (LI 4)	Moves the qi
Nei Guan (Per 6) *San Yin Jiao* (Sp 6)	Together, these points transform stasis.

Chinese medicinal formula: *Tong Qiao Huo Xue Tang* (Open the Portals & Quicken the Blood Decoction)

Ingredients: Radix Rubrus Paeoniae Lactiflorae (*Chi Shao*), 10g, Radix Ligustici Wallichii (*Chuan Xiong*), 10g, Semen Pruni Persicae (*Tao Ren*), 10g, Flos Carthami Tinctorii (*Hong Hua*), 10g, Rhizoma Acori Graminei (*Shi Chang Pu*), 10g, Tuber Curcumae (*Yu Jin*), 10g

20
Itchy Ears *(Er Yang)*

Itchy ears refers to a sensation of itchiness on the surface of the auricle or in the external auditory canal which calls for relief by scratching.

Disease causes, disease mechanisms:

I. Wind heat & damp toxins

When wind heat and damp toxins are contracted and congest in the ears, this may lead to qi and blood stagnation and stasis. If wind goes in and out through the interstices and the border of the flesh in the ears or if damp toxins with heat putrefy the flesh there, itching ears may occur.

2. Blood vacuity & wind dryness

If externally contracted wind heat and damp toxins have not been expelled but remain in the body, they may damage the qi and blood, leading to qi and blood vacuity. If there is blood vacuity, wind may be engendered. This is based on the saying, "No wind, no itching." Thus internally engendered wind may result in itching in the ears.

3. Kidney vacuity with effulgent fire

Kidney vacuity may arise from congenital insufficiency, aging, sexual taxation, etc. If there is vacuity of kidney essence or yin, yang will not be held in check properly, thus frequently leading to effulgent fire. If this fire ascends and harasses the ears, itching of the ears may be present.

Treatment based on pattern discrimination:

I. Wind heat & damp toxins

Symptoms: The patient often complains of unbearable itching in the auricles or inside the ears. Through inspection, bleeding from scratching may be found on the auricles. Superficial redness and heat are marked. Local pain is present, and, in some cases, a yellow-colored exudate may be observed. In addition, there may be fever and vexation and agitation if fire toxins are exuberant. Other symptoms may include a red tongue with slimy, yellow fur, and a rapid, forceful pulse.

Therapeutic principles: Clear heat and resolve toxins, dispel wind and eliminate dampness

Acupuncture & moxibustion:

Yi Feng (TB 17) *Jiao Sun* (TB 20)	These are local points on the triple burner channel which encircles the ear. Together, they dispel wind and eliminate dampness.
Zhong Zhu (TB 3) *Wai Guan* (TB 5)	These are distal points on the triple burner. Together, they free the flow of the channel qi, dispel wind, and dissipate heat.
Yin Ling Quan (Sp 9) *Qu Quan* (Liv 8)	Together, these points eliminate dampness and resolve toxins.

Chinese medicinal formula: Modified *Long Dan Xie Gan Tang* (Gentiana Drain the Liver Decoction)

Ingredients: Radix Gentianae Scabrae (*Long Dan Cao*), 6g, Fructus Gardeniae Jasminoidis (*Zhi Zi*), 10g, Radix Scutellariae Baicalensis (*Huang Qin*), 6g, Radix Bupleuri (*Chai Hu*), 6g, Caulis Akebiae (*Mu Tong*), 3g, Rhizoma Alismatis (*Ze Xie*), 10g, Semen Plantaginis (*Che*

Qian Zi), 10g, Cortex Radicis Dictamni Dasycarpi (*Bai Xian Pi*), 10g,
Fructus Xanthii Sibirici (*Cang Er Zi*), 10g, Fructus Kochiae Scopariae
(*Di Fu Zi*), 10g

2. Blood vacuity & wind dryness

Symptoms: Persistent itching in the auricles is the main complaint. The
auricles become coarse and cracked, and sometimes desquamation is
present. Generalized symptoms may include a sallow yellow facial
complexion, emaciation, poor appetite, fatigue, lack of strength, pale lips
and tongue, and a weak, fine pulse.

Therapeutic principles: Nourish the blood and dispel wind

Acupuncture & moxibustion:

Yi Feng (TB 17) *Wan Gu* (SI 4)	Together, these points quicken the blood and unblock the network vessels.
He Gu (LI 4) *Xue Hai* (Sp 10)	Together, these points move the qi and quicken the blood to dispel the wind, since "Wind is dispelled when the blood is quickened."
Pi Shu (Bl 20) *Ge Shu* (Bl 17)	This combination of the back transport point of the spleen and the meeting point of the blood nourishes the blood.

Chinese medicinal formula: Modified *Ba Zhen Tang* (Eight Pearls
Decoction)

Ingredients: Prepared Radix Rehmanniae (*Shu Di*),12g, Radix Angelicae
Sinensis (*Dang Gui*), 10g, Radix Albus Paeoniae Lactiflorae (*Bai Shao*),
10g, Radix Ligustici Wallichii (*Chuan Xiong*), 6g, Radix Codonopsis
Pilosulae (*Dang Shen*), 6g, Rhizoma Atractylodis Macrocephalae (*Bai
Zhu*), 6g, Sclerotium Poriae Cocos (*Fu Ling*), 10g, mix-fried Radix
Glycyrrhizae (*Zhi Gan Cao*), 6g, Periostracum Cicadae (*Chan Tui*), 15g,

Radix Ledebouriellae Divaricatae (*Fang Feng*), 10g, Fructus Kochiae Scopariae (*Di Fu Zi*), 10g

3. Kidney vacuity with effulgent fire

Symptoms: Itching in the external auditory canal may be unbearable. However, in other cases, there is only an uneasy sensation as if stimulated by a slight wind and there is no itching of the auricles. Other symptoms may include ear pain, low back pain and lack of strength, tinnitus, vertigo, a red tongue, and a fine, rapid pulse.

Therapeutic principles: Supplement the kidneys and downbear fire

Acupuncture & moxibustion:

Yi Feng (TB 17)   Together, these points harmonize the network
Ting Hui (GB 2)   vessels of the ear.

Tai Xi (Ki 3)   Together, these points nourish kidney yin in
Fu Liu (Ki 7)   order to downbear fire.

Guan Yuan (CV 4)   Supplements the kidney qi and transforms essence in order to nourish the portals of the ear

Chinese medicinal formula: *Zhi Bai Di Huang Wan* (Anemarrhena & Phellodendron Rehmannia Pills)

Ingredients: Cortex Phellodendri (*Huang Bai*), 10g, Rhizoma Anemarrhenae Asphodeloidis (*Zhi Mu*), 10g, prepared Radix Rehmanniae (*Shu Di),* 12g, Fructus Corni Officinalis (*Shan Zhu Yu*), 10g, Radix Dioscoreae Oppositae (*Shan Yao*), 10g, Rhizoma Alismatis (*Ze Xie*), 6g, Cortex Radicis Moutan (*Dan Pi*), 6g, Sclerotium Poriae Cocos (*Fu Ling*), 6g

21
Ear Pain *(Er Tong)*

Ear pain in Chinese medicine refers to pain felt by the patient in the auricles, external auditory canals, and the ear drums.

Disease causes, disease mechanisms:

I. Wind heat toxins

External heat toxins can damage the skin and muscle, cause blockage in the network vessels, and lead to qi stagnation and blood stasis. If contracted in the ears, especially when there has been an injury such as a scratch or abrasion, the network vessels there may become blocked. In that case, wind heat toxins may burn the blood and flesh and, therefore, pain occurs in the ears. Since evils may attack and remain in the auricles, external auditory canals, or middle ear, the location of the pain may be felt at any of these different sites.

2. Liver/gallbladder heat toxins

Heat toxins may come from externally contracted damp heat which brews in the channels and, over time, engenders heat toxins. They may also come from dietary irregularity which damages the spleen and leads to damp accumulation that transforms into heat and engenders heat toxins after it brews internally for some time. In addition, heat toxins may also be due to strong emotions that induces liver fire which transforms heat toxins if or when that liver fire becomes extremely exuberant. The gallbladder channel enters the ears. Therefore, if heat toxins go upward along this channel and attack the ears, they may block the network vessels there and burn the blood and flesh where it congests and brews. Hence pain may occur in the ear.

3. Qi & blood stasis and blockage

Qi and blood stasis and blockage can be the result of various factors. However, in this case, qi stagnation and blood stasis mainly come from liver/gallbladder fire which attacks above or from trauma to the ears. If qi and blood stasis blocks the network vessels in the ears, there will be pain there. This is based on the saying, "If there is pain, there is no free flow."

Treatment based on pattern discrimination:

I. Wind heat toxins

Symptoms: When pain occurs in the auricle, it is usually severe and the affected auricle is typically red in color. Pain in the external auditory canal is mainly encountered when there is an early stage sore in the ear as manifested by superficial redness, heat, and pain. This pain is exacerbated by chewing and yawning. In addition, there is red skin in the canal. Decreased auditory acuity may be present if the sore is relatively large. Pain in the middle ear is mainly seen in the early stage of contraction of external wind heat. This is accompanied by reduced auditory acuity and reddening of the eardrum. In addition to the local symptoms, generalized ones may include fever, headache, aversion to wind, fatigue, a red tongue with thin, yellow fur, and a floating, rapid pulse.

Therapeutic principles: Course wind and clear heat, resolve toxins and disperse swelling

Acupuncture & moxibustion:

Jiao Sun (TB 20)	Together, these points clear heat, resolve toxins,
Qi Mai (TB 18)	and disperse the swelling when pricked to bleed.

Qu Chi (LI 11)   Together, these points course wind and clear heat.
Wai Guan (TB 5)
He Gu (LI 4)

Additions & subtractions: For headache, add *Tai Yang* (M-HN-9). If there is reduced auditory acuity, add *Er Men* (TB 21).

Chinese medicinal formula: *Pu Ji Xiao Du Yin* (Universal Benefit Disperse Toxins Drink)

Ingredients: Fructus Arctii Lappae (*Niu Bang Zi*), 10g, Fructificatio Lasiosphaerae (*Ma Bo*), 10g, Radix Isatidis Seu Baphicacanthi (*Ban Lan Gen*), 15g, Radix Scutellariae Baicalensis (*Huang Qin*), 10g, Rhizoma Coptidis Chinensis (*Huang Lian*), 6g, Fructus Forsythiae Suspensae (*Lian Qiao*), 15g, Herba Menthae Haplocalycis (*Bo He*), 3g, Radix Scrophulariae Ningpoensis (*Xuan Shen*), 10g, Bombyx Batryticatus (*Jiang Can*), 10g, Radix Platycodi Grandiflori (*Jie Geng*), 3g, Rhizoma Cimicifugae (*Sheng Ma*), 6g, Radix Bupleuri (*Chai Hu*), 6g, Pericarpium Citri Reticulatae (*Chen Pi*), 6g, Radix Glycyrrhizae (*Gan Cao*), 3g

2. Liver/gallbladder heat toxins

Symptoms: Severe, unbearable pain in the ear, redness and swelling of the skin of the ear, red eardrum, marked decreased auditory acuity, fever, a bitter taste in the mouth, dry throat, dry stools, dark-colored urine, a red tongue with slimy, yellow fur, and a wiry, rapid pulse

Therapeutic principles: Clear the liver and drain fire

Acupuncture & moxibustion:

Yi Feng (TB 17)   Together, these points unblock the network
Er Men (TB 21)   vessels and stop pain.

Xing Jian (Liv 2)   Together, these points clear the liver and drain fire.
Qiu Xu (GB 40)
Di Wu Hui (GB 42)

Additions & subtractions: Add *Yang Ling Quan* (GB 34) for a bitter taste in the mouth. Add *Tian You* (TB 16) for reduced auditory acuity.

Chinese medicinal formula: *Long Dan Xie Gan Tang* (Gentiana Drain the Liver Decoction)

Ingredients: Radix Gentianae Scabrae (*Long Dan Cao*), 6g, Fructus Gardeniae Jasminoidis (*Zhi Zi*), 10g, Radix Scutellariae Baicalensis (*Huang Qin*), 10g, Radix Bupleuri (*Chai Hu),* 3g, Caulis Akebiae (*Mu Tong*), 3g, Rhizoma Alismatis (*Ze Xie*), 6g, Semen Plantaginis (*Che Qian Zi*), 10g, Radix Angelicae Sinensis (*Dang Gui*), 6g, uncooked Radix Rehmanniae (*Sheng Di*), 6g, Radix Glycyrrhizae (*Gan Cao*), 3g

3. Qi & blood stasis and blockage

Symptoms: The pain in the ear is radiating and unbearable. Other symptoms are dizziness, tinnitus, a dull, purple-colored tongue, and a fine, choppy pulse.

Therapeutic principles: Clear heat and drain fire, free the network vessels and unblock the portals

Acupuncture and moxibustion:

Yi Feng (TB 17)   Together, these points move the qi and quicken
Ting Hui (GB 2)   the blood.

Feng Chi (GB 20)   Together, these points clear heat in the liver and
Xing Jian (Liv 2)   gallbladder.

He Gu (LI 4)   Together, these points move the qi, quicken the
San Yin Jiao (Sp 6) blood, and transform stasis.

Chinese medicinal formula: Modified *Long Dan Xie Gan Tang* (Gentiana Drain the Liver Decoction)

Ingredients: Radix Gentianae Scabrae (*Long Dan Cao*), 6g, Fructus Gardeniae Jasminoidis (*Zhi Zi*), 10g, Radix Scutellariae Baicalensis (*Huang Qin*), 10g, Radix Bupleuri (*Chai Hu*), 6g, Caulis Akebiae (*Mu Tong*), 6g, Rhizoma Alismatis (*Ze Xie*), 6g, Semen Plantaginis (*Che Qian Zi*),10g, Radix Rubrus Paeoniae Lactiflorae (*Chi Shao*), 10g, Fructus Meliae Toosendan (*Chuan Lian Zi*), 10g, Rhizoma Corydalis Yanhusuo (*Yan Hu Suo*), 10g

22
Otopyorrhea *(Er Nei Liu Tong)*

This refers to a pussy, yellow or greenish discharge from the ear which may be either thin or thick in nature. This does not include pussy discharge from sores in the ear.

Disease causes, disease mechanisms:

Otopyorrhea mainly involves the three channels of the liver, gallbladder, and kidneys and can be roughly divided into vacuity and repletion. Replete patterns are commonly encountered in children, while the kidney yin vacuity pattern is more often seen in adults. A qi vacuity pattern may, however, be seen in small children.

I. Wind heat harassing above

Wind heat is usually contracted externally. If wind heat attacks and congests in the ears, it will smolder there and putrefy the flesh and blood in the network vessels of the ear. Therefore, otopyorrhea occurs.

2. Liver/gallbladder damp heat

Liver/gallbladder damp heat can be either contracted externally or engendered internally due to dietary irregularity which damages the spleen. This leads to accumulation of dampness and transformation of fire. It may also be due to emotional disturbance which gives rise to liver depression/qi stagnation also causing fire transformation. The gallbladder channel enters the ear. If liver/gallbladder damp heat ascends along this channel into the ears and smolders there, it will burn and putrefy the flesh and blood in the ears. Hence, otopyorrhea may occur.

3. Kidney yin vacuity with vacuity fire flaming upward

Kidney yin vacuity can be the result of constitutional yin vacuity, aging, sexual intemperance, or chronic disease (here mainly referring to prolonged otopyorrhea). If there is kidney yin vacuity, yang will not be checked properly and yin vacuity fire may flame upward along the channel. This then steams in the ear. In addition, if yin vacuity fire steams in the ears, external evils may easily invade and attack the ears. These then will transform into heat with the help of the yin vacuity fire already there. If heat smolders in the ears, it will putrefy the flesh and blood in the ears, and this may result in otopyorrhea.

4. Qi vacuity not securing

After the invasion of external evils or internal engenderment of damp heat, heat toxins may result in rupture of the eardrum. If the patient, usually a young child, is constitutionally weak, their qi may be too vacuous to secure and astringe, contain and restrain. Thus fluid flows from the portal of the ear.

Treatment based on pattern discrimination:

I. Wind heat harassing above

Symptoms: Painful distention and oppression in the ears, throbbing or stabbing pain which is made better by the discharge of the pus. Such a pussy discharge often suggests the rupture of the eardrum, and the pus is usually yellow in color. Auditory acuity may be reduced. Other symptoms are headache, fever, aversion to wind, nasal congestion and runny nose, a painful, dry throat, thirst, thin, yellow tongue fur, and a floating, rapid pulse.

Therapeutic principles: Dispel wind and clear heat, resolve the exterior with acrid, cool ingredients

Acupuncture & moxibustion:

Feng Chi (GB 20)	Together, these points clear heat and open the
Yi Feng (TB 17)	portals.
Ting Gong (SI 19)	

He Gu (LI 4)	Together, these points course wind and clear
Wai Guan (TB 5)	heat.

Shao Shang (Lu 11)	Reinforces the actions of *He Gu* and *Wai Guan* of clearing heat and resolving toxins when pricked to induce bleeding.

Additions & subtractions: For headache, add *Tai Yang* (M-HN-9) and *Shang Xing* (GV 23).

Chinese medicinal formula: Modified *Yin Qiao San* (Lonicera & Forsythia Powder)

Ingredients: Flos Lonicerae Japonicae (*Yin Hua*), 15g, Fructus Forsythiae Suspensae (*Lian Qiao*), 10g, Herba Menthae Haplocalycis (*Bo He*), 3g, Semen Praeparatus Sojae (*Dan Dou Chi*), 3g, Radix Platycodi Grandiflori (*Jie Geng*), 3g, Herba Schizonepetae Tenuifoliae (*Jing Jie*), 10g, Rhizoma Phragmitis Communis (*Lu Gen*), 10g, Folium Bambusae (*Zhu Ye*), 10g, Fructus Arctii Lappae (*Niu Bang Zi*), 15g, Radix Isatidis Seu Baphicacanthi (*Ban Lan Gen*), 20g, Radix Glycyrrhizae (*Gan Cao*), 3g

2. Liver/gallbladder damp heat

Symptoms: Abrupt onset, yellow, thick, and profuse pus, draining of the pus followed by lessening of the severe pain in the ears, fever, a bitter taste in the mouth, dry throat, headache, dry stools, dark-colored urine, slimy, yellow tongue fur, and a wiry, rapid pulse

Therapeutic principles: Clear and drain liver/gallbladder damp heat

Acupuncture & moxibustion:

Yi Feng (TB 17) *Er Men* (TB 21)	Together, these points course and regulate the channel qi in the ear to course wind, clear heat, and disinhibit the portals when needled with draining method.
Xing Jian (Liv 2) *Qu Quan* (Liv 8) *Zu Lin Qi* (GB 41)	Together, these points clear and drain damp heat of the liver and gallbladder with draining method.

Additions & subtractions: If there is high fever, add *Da Zhui* (GV 14) and *Guan Chong* (TB 1).

Chinese medicinal formula: Modified *Long Dan Xie Gan Tang* (Gentiana Drain the Liver Decoction)

Ingredients: Radix Gentianae Scabrae (*Long Dan Cao*), 6g, Radix Scutellariae Baicalensis (*Huang Qin*), 10g, Fructus Gardeniae Jasminoidis (*Zhi Zi*), 10g, Radix Bupleuri (*Chai Hu*), 6g, Caulis Akebiae (*Mu Tong*), 6g, Rhizoma Alismatis (*Ze Xie*), 6g, Semen Plantaginis (*Che Qian Zi*), 6g, Radix Angelicae Sinensis (*Dang Gui*), 6g, Radix Isatidis Seu Baphicacanthi (*Ban Lan Gen*), 20g, Radix Glycyrrhizae (*Gan Cao*), 3g

3. Kidney yin vacuity with vacuity fire flaming upward

Symptoms: On again, off again discharge of pus from the ear, thin, clear, odorless pus, dizziness, tinnitus, deafness, low back and knee aching and pain, dry mouth, vexation, tidal flushing of the face, low-grade fever, a red tongue, and a fine, rapid pulse

Therapeutic principles: Enrich yin and downbear fire

Acupuncture & moxibustion:

Lu Xi (TB 19)   Together, these points diffuse and unblock the portals
Ting Gong (SI 19)   and drain pus.

Tai Xi (Ki 3)   Together, these points enrich kidney yin and
Guan Yuan (CV 4)   downbear fire.

Additions & subtractions: Add *Fu Liu* (Ki 7) for thirst and vexation.

Chinese medicinal formula: *Zhi Bai Di Huang Wan* (Anemarrhena & Phellodendron Rehmannia Pills)

Ingredients: Cortex Phellodendri (*Huang Bai*), 15g, Rhizoma Anemarrhenae Asphodeloidis (*Zhi Mu*), 15g, prepared Radix Rehmanniae (*Shu Di*), 12g, Fructus Corni Officinalis (*Shan Zhu Yu*), 10g, Radix Dioscoreae Oppositae (*Shan Yao*), 6g, Rhizoma Alismatis (*Ze Xie*), 6g, Cortex Radicis Moutan (*Dan Pi*), 10g, Sclerotium Poriae Cocos (*Fu Ling*), 6g

4. Qi vacuity not securing

Symptoms: Chronic or enduring discharge of thin, white, odorless pus and fluids flowing from the auditory canal with no pain or inflammation. Typically, this occurs in children after an acute middle ear infection which has resulted in rupture of the eardrum. Other symptoms may include chilled limbs, a pale facial complexion, fatigue, loose stools, poor appetite, moist, thin, white tongue fur, and a deep, weak pulse.

Therapeutic principles: Fortify the spleen and boost the qi, secure, astringe, contain, and restrain

Acupuncture & moxibustion:

Yi Feng (TB 17) *Er Men* (TB 21)	Together, these points harmonize the flow of qi and blood in the ears as well as upbear the qi to secure and astringe.
Zu San Li (St 36) *Qi Hai* (CV 6)	Together, these points supplement and boost the pre- and postnatal qi.
Pi Shu (Bl 20) *Wei Shu* (Bl 21)	Together, these points fortify the spleen to engender the qi.

Chinese medicinal formula: *Huang Qi Jian Zhong Tang* (Astragalus Fortify the Center Decoction)

Ingredients: Radix Astragali Membranacei (*Huang Qi*), 10g, Maltose (*Yi Tang*), 25g, Ramulus Cinnamomi Cassiae (*Gui Zhi*), 6g, Radix Albus Paeoniae Lactiflorae (*Bai Shao*), 10g, mix-fried Radix Glycyrrhizae (*Zhi Gan Cao*), 6g, uncooked Rhizoma Zingiberis (*Sheng Jiang*), 3g, Fructus Zizyphi Jujubae (*Da Zao*), 3 pieces

23
Bleeding from the Ear *(Er Nu)*

This refers to bleeding from the external auditory canal and the middle ear. It does not cover bleeding from the auricles due to trauma.

Disease causes, disease mechanisms:

I. Upward counterflow of liver fire

Liver fire mainly arises from strong emotions. Strong emotions lead to liver depression/qi stagnation which transforms fire. If this fire ascends along the gallbladder channel to the ears, it may lead to frenetic movement of the blood. Thus there is bleeding from the ear.

2. Yin vacuity, fire effulgence

Yin vacuity fire here mainly arises from kidney yin vacuity caused by constitutional yin vacuity, sexual intemperance, chronic disease, overtaxation, or aging. If there is yin vacuity, yang will not be checked properly and this may lead to yin vacuity fire. If this fire goes up along the small intestine channel, it may burn and damage the network vessels in the ears. Therefore, bleeding from the ears may occur.

Note: The kidney channel does not directly connect with the ear. This explains why there is no swelling or painful distention of the ear which otherwise is typically caused by qi stagnation and blood stasis in the channels.

Treatment based on pattern discrimination:

I. Upward counterflow of liver fire

Symptoms: Bleeding from the ear which often occurs suddenly and with large quantity, pain in the ears, vexation and irascibility, possible distention and fullness in the chest and lateral costal regions, a bitter taste in the mouth, red eyes, headache, dark-colored urine, a red tongue, and a wiry, rapid, forceful pulse

Therapeutic principles: Clear the liver and drain heat, cool the blood and stop bleeding

Acupuncture & moxibustion:

Er Men (TB 21)   Together, these points diffuse and free the flow
Ting Hui (GB 2)   of the channel qi to stop bleeding and stop pain.
Ting Gong (SI 19)

Tai Chong (Liv 3)   Together, these points clear the liver and drain
Di Wu Hui (GB 42)   fire, downbear counterflow and stop bleeding.

Yong Quan (Ki 1)   Leads heat downward to help stop bleeding

Chinese medicinal formula: Modified *Xi Jiao Di Huang Tang* (Rhinoceros Horn & Rehmannia Decoction)

Ingredients: Cornu Bubali (*Shui Niu Jiao*), 20g, uncooked Radix Rehmanniae (*Sheng Di*), 12g, Cortex Radicis Moutan (*Dan Pi*), 12g, Radix Rubrus Paeoniae Lactiflorae (*Chi Shao*), 12g, Radix Gentianae Scabrae (*Long Dan Cao*), 6g, Herba Ecliptae Prostratae (*Han Lian Cao*), 10g

2. Yin vacuity, fire effulgence

Symptoms: Slow bleeding from the ear which is small in quantity and comes at intervals, no swelling or pain in the ears. Other symptoms may include dizziness, vertigo, heart palpitations, tinnitus, low back and knee pain and weakness, lassitude of the spirit, lack of strength, a red tongue, and a fine, rapid pulse.

Therapeutic principles: Enrich yin and downbear fire, clear heat and stop bleeding

Acupuncture & moxibustion:

Yi Feng (TB 17)	Together, these points quicken the network
Er Men (TB 21)	vessels to stop bleeding.

Yin Gu (Ki 10)	Together, these points enrich yin and downbear
Tai Xi (Ki 3)	fire to stop bleeding.
Da Dun (Liv 1)	

Remarks: For bleeding, acupuncture and moxibustion are effective. However, when the bleeding is severe, these should be combined with other appropriate therapies.

Chinese medicinal formula: Modified *Zhi Bai Di Huang Wan* (Anemarrhena & Phellodendron Rehmannia Pills)

Ingredients: Rhizoma Anemarrhenae Asphodeloidis (*Zhi Mu*), 12g, Cortex Phellodendri (*Huang Bai*), 12g, uncooked Radix Rehmanniae (*Sheng Di*), 12g, Fructus Corni Officinalis (*Shan Zhu Yu*), 10g, Radix Dioscoreae Oppositae (*Shan Yao*), 6g, Rhizoma Alismatis (*Ze Xie*), 6g, Cortex Radicis Moutan (*Dan Pi*), 6g, Sclerotium Poriae Cocos (*Fu Ling*), 6g, Radix Scrophulariae Ningpoensis (*Xuan Shen*), 10g, Herba Ecliptae Prostratae (*Han Lian Cao*), 10g

24
Epistaxis *(Bi Nu)*

Epistaxis refers to bleeding from the nostrils. Vicarious menstruation in women is not included herein.

Disease causes, disease mechanisms:

I. Wind cold remaining unresolved

When wind cold invades the body, the *tai yang* channel is often the first channel to be attacked. If this wind cold cannot be resolved through sweating and becomes depressed in the *tai yang* channel, it may ascend along the channel and harass the portal of the nose. If the correct qi is still strong enough to fight the evil and expel it from the body, bleeding from the nose may occur. In this case, this bleeding discharges the evils via the nose instead of through sweating.

2. Wind heat congesting in the lungs

When external wind heat or dry heat evils invade the body, the lungs are the first viscus to be attacked. As it is said, "The lungs open into the portal of the nose." If this heat goes upward and congests in the nose, it may burn and damage the network vessels in the nose, and hence bleeding may occur.

3. Exuberant stomach fire

Stomach fire may be due to constitutional accumulation of heat in the stomach channel or from addiction to alcoholic beverages and spicy foods. The stomach channel starts at the side of the nose, goes up to the root of the nose, and then travels down to the upper gum along the sides of the nose. If stomach fire blazes internally and flames upward along the channel to the nose, the network vessels in the nose may be burnt and damaged. Therefore, bleeding from the nose may occur.

4. Liver fire invading the lungs

Liver fire comes from frustration which gives rise to depressed liver qi or from anger which damages the liver and leads to counterflow of liver fire. When liver wood is in exuberance, it may rebel against and burn lung metal. As mentioned above, "The lungs open into the portal of the nose." If this fire counterflows upward and damages the network vessels in the nose, bleeding may occur there.

5. Spleen failing to contain the blood

Spleen qi is responsible for containing the blood and can be damaged by chronic disease, overthinking, taxation, dietary irregularity, etc. If the spleen qi becomes vacuous, the spleen may fail to contain the blood. Then the blood will move out of its vessels. Inside the nose, there are many fine and tender network vessels. If blood comes out of these vessels in the nose, bleeding from the nose will occur.

6. Kidney yin vacuity

Kidney yin vacuity may arise from congenital kidney vacuity or from sexual taxation, aging, and chronic disease. If kidney yin becomes vacuous, yin vacuity, effulgent fire may result. If this fire ascends, burns, and damages the network vessels in the nose, bleeding from the nose will occur.

7. Yin exhaustion & yang desertion

Yin exhaustion and yang desertion are mainly caused here by massive hemorrhaging. If there is great loss of blood, qi will be lost with the blood. Qi is responsible for moving, containing, and engendering the blood. If there is qi desertion, the blood will lose its containment and, therefore, nose-bleeding may occur.

Treatment based on pattern discrimination:

1. Wind cold remaining unresolved

Symptoms: A small amount of blood from the nose which is often followed by abatement of fever and which can stop spontaneously. Other symptoms may include general malaise, headache, absence of perspiration, thin tongue fur, and a floating, tight pulse.

Therapeutic principles: Promote sweating to resolve the exterior (but only if there still exists an exterior pattern of *tai yang* after spontaneous nosebleeding)

Acupuncture & moxibustion:

He Gu (LI 4) *Fu Liu* (Ki 7)	Together, these points promote sweating when *He Gu* is needled with supplementing and *Fu Liu* is needled with draining technique.
Wai Guan (TB 5) *Feng Men* (Bl 12)	Together, these points course wind and scatter cold.

Chinese medicinal formula: *Ma Huang Tang* (Ephedra Decoction)

Ingredients: Herba Ephedrae (*Ma Huang*), 10g, Ramulus Cinnamomi Cassiae (*Gui Zhi*), 6g, Semen Pruni Armeniacae (*Xing Ren*), 9g, mix-fried Radix Glycyrrhizae (*Zhi Gan Cao*), 3g

2. Wind heat congesting in the lungs

Symptoms: Bleeding from the nose with a small amount of fresh, red blood, a dry, painful nose, fever, sweating, thirst, sore throat, cough with scant phlegm, thin, white, dry tongue fur, and a floating, rapid pulse

Therapeutic principles: Course wind, clear heat, and stop bleeding

Acupuncture & moxibustion:

Feng Fu (GV 16) *Shang Xing* (GV 23)	These are points on the governing vessel which goes through the nose. Together, they clear heat and stop bleeding when needled with draining method.
Yu Ji (Lu 10)	The spring point of the lungs; clears heat from the lungs.
He Gu (LI 4)	The source point of the large intestine which has an exterior/interior relationship with the lungs; helps *Yu Ji* clear heat and also courses wind
Ying Xing (LI 20)	A local point which stops bleeding

Chinese medicinal formula: Modified *Sang Ju Yin* (Morus & Chrysanthemum Drink)

Ingredients: Flos Chrysanthemi Morifolii (*Ju Hua*), 12g, Folium Mori Albi (*Sang Ye*), 12g, Semen Pruni Armeniacae (*Xing Ren*), 6g, Herba Menthae Haplocalycis (*Bo He*), 3g, Fructus Forsythiae Suspensae (*Lian Qiao*), 10g, Radix Platycodi Grandiflori (*Jie Geng*), 10g, Rhizoma Phragmitis Communis (*Lu Gen*), 10g, Radix Glycyrrhizae (*Gan Cao*), 3g, Cortex Radicis Moutan (*Dan Pi*), 10g, Rhizoma Imperatae Cylindricae (*Bai Mao Gen*), 10g

3. Exuberant stomach fire

Symptoms: Profuse, fresh red bleeding from the nose, a dry, painful nose, vexatious thirst with a desire to drink, bad breath, swift digestion with rapid hungering, constipation, dark-colored urine, a red tongue with yellow fur, and a surging, rapid pulse

Therapeutic principles: Clear the stomach and drain fire

Acupuncture & moxibustion:

Shang Xing (GV 23)	A point on the governing vessel; clears heat to stop bleeding.
Er Jian (LI 2)	A point on the large intestine which ends at the side of the nose; clears heat in the *yang ming*.
Zhong Wan (CV 12) *Nei Ting* (St 44)	Together, these points clear and drain stomach fire.
Yin Bai (Sp 1)	Leads heat downward

Chinese medicinal formula: Modified *Yu Nu Jian* (Jade Maiden Decoction)

Ingredients: Gypsum Fibrosum (*Shi Gao*), 20g, Rhizoma Anemarrhenae Asphodeloidis (*Zhi Mu*), 12g, uncooked Radix Rehmanniae (*Sheng Di*), 12g, Tuber Ophiopogonis Japonici (*Mai Dong*), 10g, Radix Cyathulae (*Chuan Niu Xi*), 3g, Radix Et Rhizoma Rhei (*Da Huang*), 6g, Fructus Gardeniae Jasminoidis (*Zhi Zi*), 10g, Rhizoma Imperatae Cylindricae (*Bai Mao Gen*), 10g, Cacumen Biotae Orientalis (*Ce Bai Ye*), 10g

4. Liver fire invading the lungs

Symptoms: This bleeding often follows emotional disturbance and is profuse in quantity and bright red or crimson in color. The bleeding may occur repeatedly. Other symptoms may include painful distention in the head, vexation, irascibility, a bitter taste in the mouth, dry throat, fullness in the chest and lateral costal regions, red eyes, dark-colored urine, a red tongue, and a wiry, rapid pulse.

Therapeutic principles: Clear the liver, drain fire, and stop bleeding

Acupuncture & moxibustion:

Ying Xiang (LI 20)	A local point; clears heat to stop bleeding
Shao Shang (Lu 11) *Yu Ji* (Lu 10) *Wen Liu* (LI 7)	Points on the lung channel which opens into the nose; with *Wen Liu*, they clear heat in the lungs.
Da Dun (Liv 1) *Xing Jian* (Liv 2)	Points on the liver channel; together, they resolve liver depression and drain heat.

Chinese medicinal formula: Modified *Long Dan Xie Gan Tang* (Gentiana Drain the Liver Decoction)

Ingredients: Radix Gentianae Scabrae (*Long Dan Cao*), 6g, Radix Scutellariae Baicalensis (*Huang Qin*), 10g, Fructus Gardeniae Jasminoidis (*Zhi Zi*), 10g, uncooked Radix Rehmanniae (*Sheng Di*), 12g, Rhizoma Alismatis (*Ze Xie*), 3g, Semen Plantaginis (*Che Qian Zi*), 3g, Radix Bupleuri (*Chai Hu*), 3g, Radix Rubiae Cordifoliae (*Qian Cao Gen*), 10g, Flos Immaturus Sophorae Japonicae (*Huai Hua*), 10g

5. Spleen failing to contain the blood

Symptoms: The bleeding is slower in manner and typically occurs repeatedly. It is easy to stop but tends to also easily recur. The color of the blood is pale red. Other symptoms may include a pale, lusterless facial complexion, poor appetite, lassitude of the spirit, lack of strength, shortness of breath, disinclination to speak, abdominal distention, loose stools, and a soggy, fine, forceless pulse.

Therapeutic principles: Fortify the spleen, boost qi, and contain the blood

Acupuncture & moxibustion:

Pi Shu (Bl 20) *Zu San Li* (St 36)	Together, these points supplement the spleen to engender the qi and blood.
Qi Hai (CV 6)	Supplements the qi
Tai Yuan (Lu 9)	Supplements the lung qi
Shang Xing (GV 23)	Unblocks the portals and stops bleeding

Additions & subtractions: Add *Da Dun* (Liv 1) with strong moxibustion if the bleeding is severe.

Chinese medicinal formula: Modified *Gui Pi Tang* (Return the Spleen Decoction)

Ingredients: Rhizoma Atractylodis Macrocephalae (*Bai Zhu*), 10g, Radix Codonopsis Pilosulae (*Dang Shen*), 12g, Sclerotium Poriae Cocos (*Fu Ling*), 10g, Radix Astragali Membranacei (*Huang Qi*), 15g, mix-fried Radix Glycyrrhizae (*Zhi Gan Cao*), 6g, Radix Angelicae Sinensis (*Dang Gui*), 6g, Radix Auklandiae Lappae (*Mu Xiang*), 6g, Herba Agrimoniae Pilosae (*Xian He Cao*), 15g

6. Kidney yin vacuity

Symptoms: The bleeding is not profuse in quantity and is bright red in color. It occurs at irregular intervals and recurs repeatedly. Other symptoms may include thirst, dizziness, vertigo, heart palpitations, tinnitus, low back and knee pain and weakness, vexatious heat in the five hearts, tidal flushing of the face, occasional night sweats, a red tongue, and a fine, rapid pulse.

Therapeutic principles: Enrich yin, downbear fire, and stop bleeding

Acupuncture & moxibustion:

Feng Chi (GB 20)	Together, these points clear fire in the upper
Ying Xiang (LI 20)	burner when needled with draining method.

Tai Xi (Ki 3)	The source point of the kidney channel
Ran Gu (Ki 2)	The spring point of the kidney channel
	Together, these points nourish kidney yin, clear heat, and downbear fire when needled with supplementing method.

Additions & subtractions: If there are night sweats, add *Fu Liu* (Ki 7).

Chinese medicinal formula: Modified *Zhi Bai Di Huang Wan* (Anemarrhena & Phellodendron Rehmannia Pills)

Ingredients: Cortex Phellodendri (*Huang Bai*), 10g, Rhizoma Anemarrhenae Asphodeloidis (*Zhi Mu*), 10g, prepared Radix Rehmanniae (*Shu Di),* 12g, Fructus Corni Officinalis (*Shan Zhu Yu*), 10g, Radix Dioscoreae Oppositae (*Shan Yao*), 6g, Sclerotium Poriae Cocos (*Fu Ling*), 6g, Rhizoma Alismatis (*Ze Xie*), 6g, Cortex Radicis Moutan (*Dan Pi*), 6g, Herba Ecliptae Prostratae (*Han Lian Cao*), 10g, Gelatinum Corii Asini (*E Jiao*), 5g

7. Yin exhaustion & yang desertion

Symptoms: The bleeding is incessant and profuse. In severe cases, there is bleeding of the mouth, teeth, nose, ears, and skin. Other symptoms may include profuse sweating, a drained white facial complexion, an open mouth with closed eyes, counterflow frigidity of the limbs, open hands, enuresis, clouded spirt orientation, dyspnea, a pale tongue, and a faint pulse on the verge of expiry.

Therapeutic principles: Return yang and stem counterflow, boost the qi and contain the blood

Acupuncture & moxibustion:

Shen Que (CV 8)	Together, these points return yang and stem
Da Dun (Liv 1)	the desertion when stimulated with strong
Guan Yuan (CV 4)	moxibustion.

Remarks: Acupuncture and moxibustion are effective for treating bleeding. However, one should combine this treatment mode with others if the bleeding responds poorly to it alone.

Chinese medicinal formula: Modified *Shen Fu Tang* (Ginseng & Aconite Decoction) plus *Sheng Mai San* (Engender the Pulse Powder)

Ingredients: Radix Lateralis Praeparatus Aconiti Carmichaeli (*Fu Zi*), 10g, Radix Panacis Ginseng (*Ren Shen*), 15g, Fructus Schisandrae Chinensis (*Wu Wei Zi*), 12g, Tuber Ophiopogonis Japonici (*Mai Dong*), 10g, Os Draconis (*Long Gu*), 12g

25
Dry Nose *(Bi Gan)*

Dry nose refers to a lack of moisture in the nostrils.

Disease causes, disease mechanisms:

I. Exuberant heat in the lung channel

This heat mainly arises from externally contracted wind heat or from latent heat in the lung channel. If this heat goes upward and congests in the portal of the lung, *(i.e.*, the nose), it may damage the liquids there. Therefore, dryness is present in the nose.

2. Dry evils damaging the lungs

This mainly occurs in autumn when dryness is predominant. When dryness invades the body, the lungs are often the first viscus to be attacked. Dryness damages liquids. If dryness attacks the lungs, lung fluids may be damaged and thus the nose will not be sufficiently moistened. Therefore, there is dryness in the nose.

3. Exuberant stomach heat

Stomach heat can come from external evils which enter the interior and transform into heat or from dietary irregularity, especially addiction to spicy foods and alcoholic drinks. The stomach channel starts at the side of the nose. If heat goes upward along this channel and damages fluids in the nose, dryness of the nose will occur.

4. Lung yin vacuity

Lung yin vacuity mainly arises from fluid damage due to febrile diseases or from erroneous over-promotion of sweating. "The nose is the portal of the lungs." Therefore, if there is lung yin vacuity, the nose may be deprived of enough moisture. Hence dryness may occur in the nose.

5. Qi vacuity of the lungs & spleen

Qi vacuity of the lungs and spleen may be due to dietary irregularity which damages the spleen or from taxation and internal damage. The spleen is responsible for engendering the qi and blood and body fluids, while the lungs are responsible for distributing these. If there is qi vacuity of the spleen and lungs, consequently there is less qi, blood and fluids engendered and distributed to moisten and nourish the nose. Thus dryness may occur in the nose.

Treatment based on pattern discrimination:

I. Exuberant heat in the lung channel

Symptoms: Dry nostrils, burning pain, and slight itching in the nose, dry mouth and throat, cough with scant phlegm. In some severe cases, there may be fever, headache, general malaise, dry stools, and dark-colored urine. On inspection, one may see red swelling or erosion in the nostrils. The tongue is red with thin, yellow fur, and the pulse is floating and rapid or wiry and rapid.

Therapeutic principles: Clear heat and diffuse the lungs

Acupuncture & moxibustion:

Yin Xiang (LI 20) *He Liao* (LI 19)	Together, these points course and free the flow of qi in the *yang ming* channel to clear heat evils in the nose.

Zhong Fu (Lu 1)	A combination of transporting and alarm points;
Fei Shu (Bl 13)	together, they clear and drain heat in the lungs and diffuse the lungs when needled with draining method.
He Gu (LI 4)	Helps clear heat and diffuse the lungs

Chinese medicinal formula: Modified *Qing Zao Jiu Fei Tang* (Clear Dryness & Rescue the Lungs Decoction)

Ingredients: Folium Mori Albi (*Sang Ye*), 12g, Gypsum Fibrosum (*Shi Gao*), 20g, Gelatinum Corii Asini (*E Jiao*), 5g, Tuber Ophiopogonis Japonici (*Mai Dong*), 10g, Semen Pruni Armeniacae (*Xing Ren*), 10g, Folium Eriobotryae Japonicae (*Pi Pa Ye*), 10g, Rhizoma Anemarrhenae Asphodeloidis (*Zhi Mu*), 10g, Radix Glehniae Littoralis (*Bei Sha Shen*), 10g

2. Dry evils damaging the lungs

Symptoms: Dryness in the nose, nasal congestion, itchy nose, possible decreased sense of smell, dry cough with no or scant, sticky phlegm, thirst with dry lips, fever, headache, general malaise, a red tongue with thin fur and reduced liquids, and a floating, fine, rapid pulse

Therapeutic principles: Clear the lungs and moisten dryness

Acupuncture & moxibustion:

Ying Xiang (LI 20)	Together, these points clear heat and moisten
He Liao (LI 19)	dryness.
Chi Ze (Lu 5)	Together, these points nourish lung yin and clear
Fei Shu (Bl 13)	heat.
San Yin Jiao (Sp 6)	The meeting point of the three yin channels; nourishes yin.

Additions & subtractions: If the exterior pattern is pronounced, add *He Gu* (LI 4).

Chinese medicinal formula: *Sang Xing Tang* (Morus & Armeniaca Decoction)

Ingredients: Folium Mori Albi (*Sang Ye*), 12g, Semen Pruni Armeniacae (*Xing Ren*), 10g, Radix Glehniae Littoralis (*Bei Sha Shen*), 12g, Bulbus Fritillariae Cirrhosae (*Chuan Bei Mu*), 6g, Semen Praeparatus Sojae (*Dan Dou Chi*), 6g, Rhizoma Anemarrhenae Asphodeloidis (*Zhi Mu*), 10g, Tuber Ophiopogonis Japonici (*Mai Dong*), 10g

3. Exuberant stomach heat

Symptoms: Dryness with burning pain in the nose, possible nosebleeding, a dry mouth and throat, thirst with desire for cold drinks, swift digestion with rapid hungering, acid regurgitation, bad breath, clamoring stomach, constipation with dry stools, short voiding of dark-colored urine, a red tongue with yellow fur, and a slippery, rapid pulse

Therapeutic principles: Clear and drain stomach heat

Acupuncture and moxibustion:

Ying Xiang (LI 20) *He Liao* (LI 19)	Together, these points clear heat in the *yang ming* channel.
Zhong Wan (CV 12) *Nei Ting* (St 44)	Together, these points clear and drain stomach heat.
Tian Shu (St 25) *Shang Ju Xu* (St 37)	Together, these points free the stools to drain stomach fire.

Chinese medicinal formula: Modified *Qing Wei San* (Clear the Stomach Powder)

Ingredients: Uncooked Radix Rehmanniae (*Sheng Di*), 15g, Rhizoma Coptidis Chinensis (*Huang Lian*), 6g, Cortex Radicis Moutan (*Dan Pi*), 6g, Rhizoma Cimicifugae (*Sheng Ma*), 10g, Radix Angelicae Sinensis (*Dang Gui*), 6g, Rhizoma Anemarrhenae Asphodeloidis (*Zhi Mu*), 10g, Radix Et Rhizoma Rhei (*Da Huang*), 6g

4. Lung yin vacuity

Symptoms: Dryness in the nose and throat, reduced nasal mucous, cough with sticky phlegm, itchy throat, tidal fever, night sweats, vexatious heat in the five hearts, a red tongue with reduced liquids, and a fine, rapid pulse

Therapeutic principles: Nourish yin and moisten dryness

Acupuncture & moxibustion:

Ying Xiang (LI 20) *He Liao* (LI 19)	Together, these points course and regulate the channel qi.
Lie Que (Lu 7) *Fei Shu* (Bl 13)	Together, these points enrich and supplement lung yin, restore the diffusion and depuration of the lungs to moisten dryness when needled with supplementing method.
Yin Ling Quan (Sp 9)	The water point of the earth channel; it supplements the yin of lung metal when needled with supplementing method.

Chinese medicinal formula: *Bai He Gu Jin Tang* (Lily Secure Metal Decoction)

Ingredients: Bulbus Lilii (*Bai He*), 12g, uncooked Radix Rehmanniae (*Sheng Di*), 12g, Tuber Ophiopogonis Japonici (*Mai Dong*), 10g, prepared Radix Rehmanniae (*Shu Di*), 10g, Rhizoma Anemarrhenae Asphodeloidis (*Zhi Mu*), 10g, Radix Scrophulariae Ningpoensis (*Xuan*

Shen), 10g, Radix Platycodi Grandiflori (*Jie Geng*), 6g, Radix Angelicae Sinensis (*Dang Gui*), 6g, Radix Albus Paeoniae Lactiflorae (*Bai Shao*), 6g, Radix Glycyrrhizae (*Gan Cao*), 6g

5. Qi vacuity of the lungs & spleen

Symptoms: Dryness and itching in the nose, scabs on the nasal mucous membranes, a drained white facial complexion, lassitude of the spirit, lack of strength, shortness of breath, spontaneous perspiration, abdominal distention, torpid intake, loose stools, a pale tongue with thin fur, and a fine, weak pulse

Therapeutic principles: Supplement the center and boost the qi, bank earth and engender metal

Acupuncture & moxibustion:

Ying Xiang (LI 20) *Shang Xing* (GV 23)	Together, these points move the qi and blood to moisten the dryness. Moxibustion should be applied to *Shang Xing*.
Tai Yuan (Lu 9) *Zu San Li* (St 36) *Tai Bai* (Sp 3)	Together, these points bank earth and engender the metal when needled with supplementing method.

Chinese medicinal formula: *Bu Zhong Yi Qi Tang* (Supplement the Center & Boost the Qi Decoction)

Ingredients: Radix Astragali Membranacei (*Huang Qi*), 15g, Rhizoma Atractylodis Macrocephalae (*Bai Zhu*), 10g, Radix Angelicae Sinensis (*Dang Gui*), 10g, Pericarpium Citri Reticulatae (*Chen Pi*), 6g, Rhizoma Cimicifugae (*Sheng Ma*), 3g, Radix Bupleuri (*Chai Hu*), 3g, Radix Codonopsis Pilosulae (*Dang Shen*), 10g, mix-fried Radix Glycyrrhizae (*Zhi Gan Cao*), 6g

26
Nasal Itching *(Bi Yang)*

Nasal itching, as its name states, refers to an itching sensation inside the nose which calls for relief by scratching.

Disease causes, disease mechanisms:

The main disease factors leading to nasal itching are wind and heat. Itching is more severe than pain when wind is predominant, while pain is more severe if heat is predominant.

1. Wind heat invading the lungs

When wind heat invades the body, the lungs are typically the first viscus to be attacked. If such wind heat goes upward and harasses the portal of the lung, nasal itching may occur.

2. Dry heat in the lung channel

Dry heat may be directly contracted externally or it may be derived from constitutional yin vacuity. Dry heat may engender wind. If this wind goes upward and harasses the nose, nasal itching may occur.

3. Damp heat in the spleen channel

Damp heat is mainly due to spleen vacuity in turn due to dietary irregularity. It may also be from external contraction. If damp heat ascends, congests, and fumes and steams in the nose, itching may occur there.

4. Lung vacuity coupling with wind

Based on the saying, "The lungs are connected with the skin and hair and opens into the nose," when there is lung vacuity, insecurity of the defensive exterior may result. Thus wind evils may take advantage of this vacuity to invade the body. If this wind goes upward and harasses the portal of the lung, itching may occur in the nose.

Treatment based on pattern discrimination:

I. Wind heat invading the lungs

Symptoms: Itchy nose, nasal congestion, frequent sneezing, yellow nasal mucous, fever, aversion to wind, headache, sore throat, cough, a red tongue, and a floating, rapid pulse

Therapeutic principles: Course and dissipate wind heat

Acupuncture & moxibustion:

Ying Xiang (LI 20)	Unblocks the network vessels to stop itching
Lie Que (Lu 7) *He Gu* (LI 4)	A combination of source and network points; together, they course wind and clear heat, diffuse the lungs and unblock the portal of the nose.
Chi Ze (Lu 5)	Enhances the action of *Lie Que* and *He Gu*

Chinese medicinal formula: *Sang Ju Yin* (Morus & Chrysanthemum Drink)

Ingredients: Flos Chrysanthemi Morifolii (*Ju Hua*), 15g, Folium Mori Albi (*Sang Ye*), 15g, Semen Pruni Armeniacae (*Xing Ren*), 10g, Herba Menthae Haplocalycis (*Bo He*), 6g, Fructus Forsythiae Suspensae (*Lian*

Qiao), 10g, Radix Platycodi Grandiflori (*Jie Geng*), 6g, Rhizoma Phragmitis Communis (*Lu Gen*), 12g, Radix Glycyrrhizae (*Gan Cao*), 6g

2. Dry heat in the lung channel

Symptoms: Itching and dryness in the nose, a sensation of heat in the nose felt on exhalation, a dry mouth and throat, dry cough with scant phlegm which is difficult to expectorate, a red tongue with thin fur, and a rapid pulse

Therapeutic principles: Clear the lungs and moisten dryness

Acupuncture & moxibustion:

Ying Tang (M-HN-3)   Together, these points free and disinhibit the
Ying Xiang (LI 20)   portal of the nose.

Fei Shu (Bl 13)   Together, these points clear heat from the lungs
Chi Ze (Lu 5)   when needled with draining method.

Fu Liu (Ki 7)   Nourishes yin to moisten dryness

Chinese medicinal formula: Modified *Qing Zao Jiu Fei Tang* (Clear Dryness & Rescue the Lungs Decoction)

Ingredients: Folium Mori Albi (*Sang Ye*), 12g, Gypsum Fibrosum (*Shi Gao*), 20g, Tuber Ophiopogonis Japonici (*Mai Dong*), 10g, Rhizoma Anemarrhenae Asphodeloidis (*Zhi Mu*), 10g, Radix Glehniae Littoralis (*Bei Sha Shen*), 10g, Gelatinum Corii Asini (*E Jiao*), 5g, Semen Pruni Armeniacae (*Xing Ren*), 10g, Folium Eriobotryae Japonicae (*Pi Pa Ye*), 10g, Radix Glycyrrhizae (*Gan Cao*), 6g

3. Damp heat in the spleen channel

Symptoms: Itching in the nose with yellowish water running out, in some cases, redness, swelling, and ulceration in the nose, distention and fullness in the stomach and abdomen, reduced food intake, loose stools, slimy, yellow tongue fur, and a soggy, rapid pulse

Therapeutic principles: Clear heat and dispel dampness

Acupuncture & moxibustion:

Shang Xing (GV 23) *Ying Xiang* (LI 20)	Together, these points clear heat and dispel dampness in the portal of the nose.
Nei Ting (St 44) *Yin Ling Quan* (Sp 9)	Together, these points clear heat and disinhibit dampness.

Additions & subtractions: If dampness is predominant, add *Feng Long* (St 40). If heat is predominant, add *Jie Xi* (St 41).

Chinese medicinal formula: Modified *Chu Shi Tang* (Eliminate Dampness Decoction)

Ingredients: Talcum (*Hua Shi*), 10g, Semen Plantaginis (*Che Qian Zi*), 10g, Radix Scutellariae Baicalensis (*Huang Qin*), 6g, Rhizoma Coptidis Chinensis (*Huang Lian*), 6g, Caulis Akebiae (*Mu Tong*), 3g, Sclerotium Poriae Cocos (*Fu Ling*), 10g, Pericarpium Citri Reticulatae (*Chen Pi*), 10g, Fructus Forsythiae Suspensae (*Lian Qiao*), 6g, Fructus Citri Aurantii (*Zhi Ke*), 6g, Herba Agastachis Seu Pogostemi (*Huo Xiang*), 10g

4. Lung vacuity coupling with wind

Symptoms: Paroxysmal itching in the nose, suffering due to frequent sneezing, spontaneous perspiration, lack of strength, a drained white facial complexion, a pale tongue with thin fur, and a floating, weak pulse

Therapeutic principles: Supplement the lungs and course wind

Acupuncture & moxibustion:

Shang Xing (GV 23) *Ying Xiang* (LI 20)	Together, these points course wind to stop itching.
Tai Yuan (Lu 9) *Tai Bai* (Sp 3) *He Gu* (LI 4)	Together, these points bank earth and engender the metal to secure the exterior.

Chinese medicinal formula: *Yu Ping Feng San* (Jade Windscreen Powder)

Ingredients: Radix Astragali Membranacei (*Huang Qi*), 25g, Rhizoma Atractylodis Macrocephalae (*Bai Zhu*), 15g, Radix Ledebouriellae Divaricatae (*Fang Feng*), 12g

27
Nose Pain *(Bi Tong)*

This refers to the pain occurring in the region of the nose. Nose pain can occur along with swelling of the nose, dryness in the nose, etc. Below, we deal only with nose pain when it is the major complaint of the patient.

Disease causes, disease mechanisms:

I. Congestion & stagnation of wind, cold & dampness

If external wind, cold, and/or damp evils invade the body, they may congest and stagnate in the channels and network vessels. If this congestion takes place in the network vessels in the nose, pain will occur there, since, "If there is no free flow, there is pain."

2. Wind heat congesting in the lungs

If wind heat evils invade the body, the lungs are typically the first viscus to be attacked. In that case, the wind heat congests in the lungs. Because "The nose is the portal of the lungs," if this wind heat ascends and congests in the network vessels in the nose, pain may occur there.

3. Exuberant heat of the lungs & stomach

Exuberant heat of the lungs and stomach mainly results from addiction to alcohol and spicy foods or from externally contracted fire evils. The stomach channel starts at the sides of the nose and the lungs open into the nose. If fire or heat goes up along the channel, harasses the nose, and congests in the network vessels there, blockage will occur in the nose. Therefore, nose pain may be present.

Treatment based on pattern discrimination:

1. Congestion & stagnation of wind, cold & dampness

Symptoms: Slight pain in the nostrils, nasal congestion, runny nose with clear mucous, slight aversion to wind and cold, fever, fullness in the stomach, torpid intake, abdominal distention, loose stools, thin, possibly slimy, white tongue fur, and a floating, rapid pulse

Therapeutic principles: Dispel wind, transform dampness, and scatter cold

Acupuncture & moxibustion:

Chi Ze (Lu 5)	Together, these points diffuse lungs to transform
Lie Que (Lu 7)	dampness, course wind, and scatter cold.
He Gu (LI 4)	Together, these points course and free the *yang ming*
Ying Xiang (LI 20)	channel qi to stop pain.

Chinese medicinal formula: Modified *Huo Xiang Zheng Qi San* (Agastaches Correct the Qi Powder)

Ingredients: Herba Agastachis Seu Pogostemi (*Huo Xiang*), 10g, Folium Perillae Frutescentis (*Zi Su Ye*), 10g, Radix Angelicae Dahuricae (*Bai Zhi*), 10g, Pericarpium Arecae Catechu (*Da Fu Pi*), 6g, Sclerotium Poriae Cocos (*Fu Ling*), 10g, Rhizoma Atractylodis Macrocephalae (*Bai Zhu*), 10g, Radix Puerariae (*Ge Gen*), 10g, Rhizoma Pinelliae Ternatae (*Ban Xia*), 10g, Pericarpium Citri Reticulatae (*Chen Pi*), 6g, Cortex Magnoliae Officinalis (*Hou Po*), 6g, Radix Platycodi Grandiflori (*Jie Geng*), 6g, Fructus Xanthii Sibirici (*Cang Er Zi*), 10g, mix-fried Radix Glycyrrhizae (*Zhi Gan Cao*), 3g

2. Wind heat congesting in the lungs

Symptoms: Burning pain in the nostrils, redness and swelling in the nose, runny nose with turbid mucous, fever, headache, thirst, sore throat, cough with yellow phlegm, a red tongue with thin, possibly slightly yellow fur, and a floating, rapid pulse

Therapeutic principles: Dispel wind and clear heat

Acupuncture & moxibustion:

Zhong Fu (Lu 1) *Fei Shu* (Bl 13)	Together, these points clear and drain heat in the lungs.
Lie Que (Lu 7) *He Gu* (LI 4)	Together, these points dispel wind and resolve the exterior.
Ying Xiang (LI 20)	Unblocks the network vessels to stop the pain

Additions & subtractions: If there is high fever, add *Da Zhui* (GV 14).

Chinese medicinal formula: Modified *Sang Ju Yin* (Morus & Chrysanthemum Drink)

Ingredients: Flos Chrysanthemi Morifolii (*Ju Hua*), 12g, Folium Mori Albi (*Sang Ye*), 12g, Semen Pruni Armeniacae (*Xing Ren*), 6g, Herba Menthae Haplocalycis (*Bo He*), 6g, Fructus Forsythiae Suspensae (*Lian Qiao*), 10g, Radix Platycodi Grandiflori (*Jie Geng*), 10g, Fructus Xanthii Sibirici (*Cang Er Zi*), 10g, Radix Puerariae (*Ge Gen*), 10g, Radix Glycyrrhizae (*Gan Cao*), 6g

3. Exuberant heat of the lungs & stomach

Symptoms: Severe pain often occurring in the lower part of the nostrils or in the septum which is exacerbated by pressure. In some cases, slight bleeding may be present. Other symptoms may include thirst, a dry throat, constipation, dark-colored urine, yellow tongue fur, and a rapid pulse.

Therapeutic principles: Drain the lungs and clear the stomach

Acupuncture & moxibustion:

Chi Ze (Lu 5)	Together, these points clear and drain heat in the
Qu Chi (Lu 11)	lungs and stomach when needled with draining
Nei Ting (St 44)	method.
Ying Xiang (LI 20)	Together, these points clear heat and unblock the
He Liao (LI 19)	network vessels in the nose to stop pain.
Fu Liu (Ki 7)	Protects yin to avoid damage to the liquids

Chinese medicinal formula: Modified *Qing Wei San* (Clear the Stomach Powder)

Ingredients: Uncooked Radix Rehmanniae (*Sheng Di*), 10g, Rhizoma Coptidis Chinensis (*Huang Lian*), 6g, Rhizoma Cimicifugae (*Sheng Ma*), 10g, Cortex Radicis Moutan (*Dan Pi*), 6g, Radix Et Rhizoma Rhei (*Da Huang*), 6g, Radix Scutellariae Baicalensis (*Huang Qin*), 6g, Radix Glycyrrhizae (*Gan Cao*), 6g

28
Runny Nose *(Bi Liu Ti)*

Runny nose refers to running downward of excessive mucous secretions from the nose.

Disease causes, disease mechanisms:

I. Wind cold invading the lungs

If wind cold invades the body, this will fetter the exterior and lead to non-diffusion of the lungs. This is based on the sayings, "The lungs govern the skin and hair" and "The lungs open into the nose." If there is non-diffusion of the lungs, the qi dynamic will not be free in the nose and thus the flow of qi and blood and fluids will be inhibited there. Hence there is runny nose.

2. Wind heat invading the lungs

If wind heat invades the body, non-diffusion of lung qi will typically result. With non-diffusion of lung qi, the nose will be inhibited. If fluids in the nose are fumed and steamed by this wind heat, runny nose may occur.

3. Spleen/stomach damp heat

Damp heat mainly arises from addiction to alcohol and fatty and/or sweet foods which engender damp heat internally. If this damp heat depresses and encumbers the spleen and stomach, resulting in abnormal movement and transformation of the spleen and stomach, the clear qi will not be upborne, while the turbid yin will not be downborne. The spleen has an exterior/interior relationship with the stomach and the stomach channel starts at the side of the nose. Therefore, if damp heat goes up along the channel into the nose and congests there, runny nose may result.

4. Qi vacuity

The qi may become vacuous due to chronic disease, taxation, overthinking, etc. If lung qi is vacuous, water may be inhibited. In that case, water dampness may flood and run through the nose. If spleen qi is vacuous, water dampness will accumulate internally, and runny nose may occur when this water dampness floods upward.

Treatment based on pattern discrimination:

I. Wind cold invading the lungs

Symptoms: Profuse, clear discharge from the nose accompanied by nasal congestion, frequent sneezing, fever, aversion to wind and cold, headache, cough, absence of sweating, a pale red tongue with thin, white fur, and a floating, tight pulse

Therapeutic principles: Resolve the exterior with warm, acrid ingredients, course wind and scatter cold

Acupuncture & moxibustion:

Shang Xing (GV 23) *Ying Xiang* (LI 20)	Together, these points diffuse and unblock the portal of the nose. Moxibustion should be used on the point *Shang Xing*.
Feng Men (Bl 12) *Lie Que* (Lu 7)	Together, these points course wind, scatter cold, and resolve the exterior.

Chinese medicinal formula: Modified *Cang Er Zi San* (Xanthium Powder)

Ingredients: Herba Ephedrae (*Ma Huang*), 10g, Herba Schizonepetae Tenuifoliae (*Jing Jie*), 10g, Fructus Xanthii Sibirici (*Cang Er Zi*), 10g, Flos Magnoliae Liliflorae (*Xin Yi Hua*), 10g, Herba Agastachis Seu Pogostemi (*Huo Xiang*), 10g, Radix Angelicae Dahuricae (*Bai Zhi*), 10g, Herba Cum Radice Asari (*Xi Xin*), 3g

2. Wind heat invading the lungs

Symptoms: Profuse, thick, yellow nasal discharge, in severe cases, pain, redness, and swelling in and around the nostrils, headache, fever, aversion to wind, cough, sweating, a red tongue with white fur, and a floating, rapid pulse

Therapeutic principles: Resolve the exterior with cool, acrid ingredients, course wind, clear heat, and unblock the portals

Acupuncture & moxibustion:

Ying Xiang (LI 20)	Together, these points course wind, dissipate
Ying Tang (M-HM-3)	heat, and unblock the portals.

Chi Ze (Lu 5)	Together, these points clear heat, diffuse the
Yu Ji (Lu 10)	lungs, and resolve the exterior.
He Gu (LI 4)	

Chinese medicinal formula: Modified *Cang Er Zi San* (Xanthium Powder)

Ingredients: Folium Mori Albi (*Sang Ye*), 10g, Flos Chrysanthemi Morifolii (*Ju Hua*), 10g, Herba Menthae Haplocalycis (*Bo He*), 6g, Radix Puerariae (*Ge Gen*), 10g, Fructus Xanthii Sibirici (*Cang Er Zi*),

10g, Flos Magnoliae Liliflorae (*Xin Yi Hua*), 10g, Radix Angelicae Dahuricae (*Bai Zhi*), 10g

3. Spleen/stomach damp heat

Symptoms: Runny nose with profuse, yellow, turbid discharge. In some cases, the patient complains that the nasal discharge counterflows into the throat. This discharge often smells fishy and offensive. Nasal congestion is serious and diminished sense of smell is often present. Other symptoms may include headache with heavy-headedness, fullness in the stomach, torpid intake, a bitter taste and stickiness in the mouth, no desire for liquids, dark-colored urine, a red tongue with slimy, yellow fur, and a slippery, rapid or soggy, rapid pulse.

Therapeutic principles: Clear heat, disinhibit dampness, and unblock the portals

Acupuncture & moxibustion:

Ying Xiang (LI 20) *He Liao* (LI 19)	Together, these points unblock the portals of the nose.
Nei Ting (St 44) *Jie Xi* (St 41) *Yin Ling Quan* (Sp 9)	Together, these points clear and disinhibit damp heat in the spleen and stomach.

Chinese medicinal formulas:

If dampness is predominant: Modified *Jia Wei Si Ling San* (Added Flavors Four [Ingredients] Poria Powder)

Ingredients: Sclerotium Poriae Cocos (*Fu Ling*), 10g, Sclerotium Polypori Umbellati (*Zhu Ling*), 10g, Rhizoma Alismatis (*Ze Xie*), 10g, Rhizoma Atractylodis Macrocephalae (*Bai Zhu*), 10g, Cortex Magnoliae Officinalis (*Hou Po*), 6g, Pericarpium Citri Reticulatae (*Chen Pi*), 6g,

Herba Agastachis Seu Pogostemi (*Huo Xiang*), 10g, Fructus Xanthii Sibirici (*Cang Er Zi*), 10g

If heat is predominant: Modified *Huang Qin Hua Shi Tang* (Scutellaria & Talcum Decoction)

Ingredients: Radix Scutellariae Baicalensis (*Huang Qin*), 10g, Talcum (*Hua Shi*), 10g, Fructus Cardamomi (*Bai Dou Kou*), 6g, Pericarpium Arecae Catechu (*Da Fu Pi*), 10g, Sclerotium Polypori Umbellati (*Zhu Ling*), 10g, Sclerotium Poriae Cocos (*Fu Ling*), 10g, Herba Cum Radice Houttuyniae Cordatae (*Yu Xing Cao*), 10g, Herba Agastachis Seu Pogostemi (*Huo Xiang*), 10g, Fructus Xanthii Sibirici (*Cang Er Zi*), 10g

4. Qi vacuity

Symptoms: Runny nose, a clear, watery discharge, in prolonged cases, a whitish, malodorous discharge, nasal congestion, runny nose precipitated by cold or on exposure to some allergic agent. Other symptoms may include shortness of breath, disinclination to speak, fatigue, lack of strength, possible fullness in the stomach, torpid intake, loose stools, a fat, pale tongue with white fur, and a slow, forceless pulse.

Therapeutic principles: Boost the lungs and secure the exterior or supplement the lungs and boost the spleen

Acupuncture & moxibustion:

Ying Xiang (LI 20)	Together, these points warm and unblock the
Bai Hui (GV 20)	portal to the nose. Use strong moxibustion for
Shang Xing (GV 23)	the points *Bai Hui* and *Shang Xing*.

Tai Yuan (Lu 9)	Together, these points bank earth and engender
Zu San Li (St 36)	the metal to boost the qi and secure the exterior
He Gu (LI 4)	when needled with supplementing method.

Chinese medicinal formulas:

If lung qi vacuity is predominant: *Yu Ping Feng San* (Jade Wind Screen Powder) plus *Cang Er Zi San* (Xanthium Powder)

Ingredients: Radix Astragali Membranacei (*Huang Qi*), 15g, Rhizoma Atractylodis Macrocephalae (*Bai Zhu*), 12g, Radix Ledebouriellae Divaricatae (*Fang Feng*), 6g, Fructus Xanthii Sibirici (*Cang Er Zi*), 10g, Flos Magnoliae Liliflorae (*Xin Yi Hua*), 10g, Radix Angelicae Dahuricae (*Bai Zhi*), 10g, Herba Menthae Haplocalycis (*Bo He*), 6g

If there is qi vacuity of both the spleen and lungs: Modified *Bu Zhong Yi Qi Tang* (Supplement the Center & Boost the Qi Decoction)

Ingredients: Radix Astragali Membranacei (*Huang Qi*), 15g, Rhizoma Atractylodis Macrocephalae (*Bai Zhu*), 10g, Radix Codonopsis Pilosulae (*Dang Shen*), 10g, Pericarpium Citri Reticulatae (*Chen Pi*), 10g, Rhizoma Cimicifugae (*Sheng Ma*), 3g, Radix Bupleuri (*Chai Hu*), 3g, Fructus Xanthii Sibirici (*Cang Er Zi*), 10g, Flos Magnoliae Liliflorae (*Xin Yi Hua*), 10g, mix-fried Radix Glycyrrhizae (*Zhi Gan Cao*), 6g

29
Nasal Congestion *(Bi Se)*

Nasal congestion refers to a feeling of difficulty breathing through the nose due to obstruction.

Disease causes, disease mechanisms:

I. Wind cold

If wind cold invades the body, it will fetter the exterior and leads to non-diffusion of lung qi. As it is said, "The lungs open into the portal of the nose." With non-diffusion of lung qi, wind cold may congest in the nose, causing blockage in the network vessels there and give rise to nasal congestion.

2. Wind heat

Wind heat invades the body mainly through the mouth and nose. If there is invasion of wind heat, the depurative function of the lungs is impaired. As a result, wind heat evils may remain in the nose and lead to inhibition of the flow of qi and blood, resulting in blockage there. Therefore, nasal congestion occurs.

3. Depressive heat in the lung channel

Depressive heat mainly derives from externally contracted wind heat or wind cold which has transformed into heat over time. If this heat goes upward and congests in the nose, nasal congestion may occur.

4. Qi vacuity of the lungs & spleen

Qi vacuity may arise from chronic disease, taxation, overthinking, or dietary irregularity. "The lung opens into the nose." Therefore, the free flow of air through the nose relies on harmonious lung qi. If the lung qi becomes vacuous, insecurity of defensive yang will exist, making the body susceptible to the invasion of external evils. When such external evils invade the body, the depuration of the lungs will be impaired and the invading evils may stagnate in the nose, leading to congestion of the nose. Spleen qi is responsible for upbearing the clear qi and downbearing the turbid. If the spleen qi becomes vacuous, the clear qi cannot be upborne, while the turbid is not downborne. If the turbid stagnates in the nose and blocks the network vessels there, nasal congestion will occur.

5. Qi stagnation & blood stasis

"In enduring disease, evils enter the network vessels." If there is repeated invasion of external evils into the nose, the correct qi will become weaker and weaker. Little by little, these evils will enter and remain in the network vessels in the nose. Consequently, blockage will be brought about, leading to qi stagnation and blood stasis in the nose. Therefore, nasal congestion may occur.

Treatment based on pattern discrimination:

I. Wind cold

Symptoms: Acute nasal congestion accompanied by runny nose with clear mucous, sneezing, fever, aversion to cold, thin, white tongue fur, and a floating or floating, tight pulse

Therapeutic principles: Course wind, scatter cold, and unblock the portals

Acupuncture & moxibustion:

Shang Xing (GV 23)   Together, these points course wind, scatter cold,
Ying Xiang (LI 20)   and unblock the portals.

Lie Que (Lu 7)   Together, these points course wind and scatter
He Gu (LI 4)   cold, diffuse the lungs and resolve the exterior.
Wai Guan (TB 5)

Chinese medicinal formula: Modified *Xin Yi San* (Flos Magnoliae Powder)

Ingredients: Flos Magnoliae Liliflorae (*Xin Yi Hua*), 12g, Herba Cum Radice Asari (*Xi Xin*), 3g, Radix Et Rhizoma Ligustici Chinensis (*Gao Ben*), 6g, Radix Angelicae Dahuricae (*Bai Zhi*), 10g, Radix Ligustici Wallichii (*Chuan Xiong*), 10g, Radix Ledebouriellae Divaricatae (*Fang Feng*), 10g, Fructus Xanthii Sibirici (*Cang Er Zi*), 10g, Herba Agastachis Seu Pogostemi (*Huo Xiang*), 10g, mix-fried Radix Glycyrrhizae (*Zhi Gan Cao*), 3g

2. Wind heat

Symptoms: Acute, often serious nasal congestion, runny nose with yellow mucous, fever, headache, aversion to wind, sweating, thirst, sore throat, thin, yellow tongue fur, and a floating, rapid pulse

Therapeutic principles: Course wind, clear heat, and unblock the portals

Acupuncture & moxibustion:

Ying Tang (M-HM-3)   Together, these points course and free the channel
Ying Xiang (LI 20)   qi to unblock the portals.

He Gu (LI 4)   Together, these points course wind, clear heat,
Da Zhui (GV 14)   and resolve the exterior when needled with
Qu Chi (LI 11)   draining method.

Chinese medicinal formula: Modified *Cang Er Zi San* (Xanthium Powder)

Ingredients: Fructus Xanthii Sibirici (*Cang Er Zi*), 10g, Flos Magnoliae Liliflorae (*Xin Yi Hua*), 10g, Radix Angelicae Dahuricae (*Bai Zhi*), 10g, Herba Menthae Haplocalycis (*Bo He*), 6g, Flos Chrysanthemi Morifolii (*Ju Hua*), 10g, Folium Mori Albi (*Sang Ye*), 10g, Fructus Forsythiae Suspensae (*Lian Qiao*), 10g, Flos Lonicerae Japonicae (*Yin Hua*), 10g

3. Depressive heat in the lung channel

Symptoms: Typically chronic, persistent or intermittent nasal congestion, runny nose with sticky, yellow mucous, distention in the head, diminished sense of smell, reduced memory power, a red tongue with slightly yellow fur, a wiry, rapid pulse

Therapeutic principles: Course wind and clear heat, drain pus and unblock the portals

Acupuncture & moxibustion:

Ying Xiang (LI 20) *Ying Tang* (M-HN-3)	Together, these points drain pus and open the portals when needled with draining method.
Zhong Fu (Lu 1) *Fei Shu* (Bl 13)	A combination of transporting and alarm points; together, they drain heat from the lungs when needled with draining method.
He Gu (LI 4)	Courses wind and also helps clear heat

Chinese medicinal formula: Modified *Cang Er Zi San* (Xanthium Powder)

Ingredients: Fructus Xanthii Sibirici (*Cang Er Zi*), 10g, Flos Magnoliae Liliflorae (*Xin Yi Hua*), 10g, Radix Angelicae Dahuricae (*Bai Zhi*), 10g,

Herba Menthae Haplocalycis (*Bo He*), 6g, Herba Cum Radice Houttuyniae Cordatae (*Yu Xing Cao*), 10g, Radix Scutellariae Baicalensis (*Huang Qin*), 10g, Radix Platycodi Grandiflori (*Jie Geng*), 10g

4. Qi vacuity of the lungs & spleen

Symptoms: Persistent nasal congestion which can alternate from one side to the other and is better or worse from time to time, exacerbation often related to exposure to cold. Other symptoms may include diminished sense of smell, dry, itchy nose, thin, white tongue fur, and a fine pulse.

Therapeutic principles: Supplement the lungs, boost the spleen, and unblock the portals

Acupuncture & moxibustion:

Ying Xiang (LI 20)	Together, these points warm and unblock the
Bai Hui (GV 20)	portals of the nose. Use moxibustion on *Bai Hui*
Shang Xing (GV 23)	and *Shang Xing*.

Fei Shu (Bl 13)	Together, these points bank earth and engender
Pi Shu (Bl 20)	the metal to boost the qi.

Chinese medicinal formulas:

If lung qi is predominantly vacuous: Modified *Wen Fei Zhi Liu Dan* (Warm the Lungs & Stop Flow Elixir)

Ingredients: Radix Panacis Ginseng (*Ren Shen*), 6g, Radix Astragali Membranacei (*Huang Qi*), 15g, Herba Schizonepetae Tenuifoliae (*Jing Jie*), 6g, Herba Cum Radice Asari (*Xi Xin*), 3g, Radix Platycodi Grandiflori (*Jie Geng*), 6g, Fructus Xanthii Sibirici (*Cang Er Zi*), 10g

If spleen qi is predominantly vacuous: Modified *Shen Ling Bai Zhu San* (Ginseng, Poria & Actractylodes Powder)

Ingredients: Radix Panacis Ginseng (*Ren Shen*), 6g, Sclerotium Poriae Cocos (*Fu Ling*), 10g, Rhizoma Atractylodis Macrocephalae (*Bai Zhu*), 10g, Radix Dioscoreae Oppositae (*Shan Yao*), 10g, Semen Nelumbinis Nuciferae (*Lian Zi*), 10g, Radix Platycodi Grandiflori (*Jie Geng*), 6g, Fructus Amomi (*Sha Ren*), 6g, Herba Cum Radice Asari (*Xi Xin*), 3g, Fructus Xanthii Sibirici (*Cang Er Zi*), 10g, mix-fried Radix Glycyrrhizae (*Zhi Gan Cao*), 3g

5. Qi stagnation & blood stasis

Symptoms: Persistent nasal congestion accompanied by runny nose with profuse, possibly thick, yellow mucous, diminished sense of smell, cough with profuse phlegm, tinnitus or deafness, a red tongue with static spots, and a wiry, fine pulse

Therapeutic principles: Harmonize the qi and blood, move stagnation and transform stasis

Acupuncture & moxibustion:

Ying Xiang (LI 20)	Together, these points transform stasis and
Ying Tang (M-HM-3)	unblock the portals when pricked to induce bleeding.
He Gu (LI 4)	Together, these points move the qi and quicken
San Yin Jiao (Sp 6)	the blood.
Pi Shu (Bl 20)	Engenders the blood in order to quicken the blood

Chinese medicinal formula: Modified *Tong Qiao Huo Xue Tang* (Open the Portals & Quicken the Blood Decoction)

Ingredients: Radix Rubrus Paeoniae Lactiflorae (*Chi Shao*), 10g, Radix Ligustici Wallichii (*Chuan Xiong*), 10g, Semen Pruni Persicae (*Tao Ren*), 10g, Flos Carthami Tinctorii (*Hong Hua*), 10g, Herba Cum Radice Asari (*Xi Xin*), 3g, Flos Magnoliae Liliflorae (*Xin Yi Hua*), 10g, Fructus Xanthii Sibirici (*Cang Er Zi*), 10g

30
Loss of Smell *(Shi Xiu)*

This refers to the loss or impairment of the sense of smell. In clinical practice, it is closely related to nasal congestion and runny nose.

Disease causes, disease mechanisms:

I. Wind heat in the lung channel

Wind heat in the lung channel mainly arises from externally contracted wind heat or wind cold which enters the interior and transforms into heat. If wind heat leads to non-diffusion of lung qi, loss of smell may occur since there is no ability to smell if lung qi does not diffuse. If wind heat goes upward and congests in the nose, loss of smell will also occur.

2. Depressive heat in the gallbladder

This heat may come from emotional disturbance, such as frustration or strong anger, or from externally contracted heat evil which enters the interior. If depressive heat transforms into fire and goes upward to harass the portals of the nose, loss of smell may occur.

3. Damp heat in the spleen channel

Damp heat may be the result of externally contracted damp heat or dampness which enters into the interior and transforms into heat. It may also be from dietary irregularity leading to accumulation of dampness which, over time, engenders damp heat. If damp heat encumbers the spleen and leads to failure of the spleen to upbear clear qi and downbear the turbid, turbid yin will congest in the nose and thus loss of smell may occur.

4. Dual vacuity of the lungs & spleen

Such dual vacuity may be the result of chronic disease, taxation, overthinking, or dietary irregularity. The spleen is the earth viscus, while the lungs are the metal viscus. If there is spleen vacuity, the mother, earth, cannot engender the son, metal. In that case, the spleen will fail to move the essence of grains and water to the lungs, leading to lung vacuity. "The lungs open into the portal of the nose." Hence, if there is lung vacuity, the nose may not be sufficiently nourished. Therefore, loss of smell may occur.

5. Qi stagnation & blood stasis

Qi stagnation and blood stasis mainly develop from the enduring existence of evils in the nose or from traumatic injury to the area of the nose. If there is qi stagnation and blood stasis, the nose cannot receive enough nourishment. Therefore, loss of smell may occur.

6. Dual vacuity of qi & blood

This vacuity may be from constitutional vacuity, great loss of blood, spleen/stomach vacuity weakness, etc. The sense of smell relies on the nourishment of the qi and blood. If there is dual vacuity of qi and blood, the nose will be deprived of sufficient nourishment. Therefore, loss of smell may occur.

Treatment based on pattern discrimination:

I. Wind heat in the lung channel

Symptoms: Diminished sense of smell often accompanied by nasal congestion, runny nose with yellow nasal mucous, fever, cough with profuse phlegm, a red tongue with thin, yellow fur, and a floating, rapid pulse

Therapeutic principles: Dispel wind and clear heat

Acupuncture & moxibustion:

Ying Xiang (LI 20) *Tong Tian* (Bl 7)	Together, these points diffuse and unblock the portals of the nose.
He Gu (LI 4) *Chi Ze* (Lu 5) *Zhong Fu* (Lu 1)	Together, these points course wind and clear heat in the lungs.

Chinese medicinal formula: Modified *Cang Er Zi San* (Xanthium Powder)

Ingredients: Fructus Xanthii Sibirici (*Cang Er Zi*), 10g, Flos Magnoliae Liliflorae (*Xin Yi Hua*), 10g, Radix Angelicae Dahuricae (*Bai Zhi*), 10g, Herba Menthae Haplocalycis (*Bo He*), 6g, Flos Chrysanthemi Morifolii (*Ju Hua*), 10g, Folium Mori Albi (*Sang Ye*), 10g, Fructus Forsythiae Suspensae (*Lian Qiao*), 10g, Flos Lonicerae Japonicae (*Yin Hua*), 10g

2. Depressive heat in the gallbladder channel

Symptoms: Diminished sense of smell accompanied by runny nose with yellow, turbid, malodorous nasal mucous. However, the capacity to smell is restored when nasal congestion is relieved. Other symptoms may include fever, headache, a bitter taste in the mouth, dry throat, profuse phlegm, lack of strength, a red tongue with yellow fur, and a wiry, rapid pulse.

Therapeutic principles: Clear the gallbladder and drain heat

Acupuncture & moxibustion:

Ying Xiang (LI 20)	Courses and frees the channel qi in the nose to unblock the portals
Qiu Xu (GB 40) *Feng Chi* (GB 20) *Xing Jian* (Liv 2)	Together, these points clear and drain depressive heat in the gallbladder.

Chinese medicinal formula: Modified *Long Dan Xie Gan Tang* (Gentiana Drain the Liver Decoction)

Ingredients: Radix Gentianae Scabrae (*Long Dan Cao*), 6g, Fructus Gardeniae Jasminoidis (*Zhi Zi*), 10g, Radix Scutellariae Baicalensis (*Huang Qin*), 10g, Radix Bupleuri (*Chai Hu*), 6g, Rhizoma Alismatis (*Ze Xie*), 6g, Herba Cum Radice Houttuyniae Cordatae (*Yu Xing Cao*), 10g, Fructus Xanthii Sibirici (*Cang Er Zi*), 10g, Semen Plantaginis (*Che Qian Zi*), 10g, Radix Glycyrrhizae (*Gan Cao*), 3g

3. Damp heat in the spleen channel

Symptoms: Diminished or no sense of smell, runny nose with yellow, sticky, malodorous nasal mucous, nasal congestion, headache, heavy-headedness, cough with yellow phlegm, distention and oppression in the stomach and abdomen, poor appetite, nonfree-flowing defecation with sticky stools, dark-colored urine, a red tongue with slimy, yellow fur, and a slippery, rapid pulse

Therapeutic principles: Clear and disinhibit dampness and heat

Acupuncture & moxibustion:

Ying Xiang (LI 20) *He Liao* (LI 19)	Together, these points clear heat in the *yang ming* channel.

Nei Ting (St 44)   Together, these points clear and disinhibit
San Yin Jiao (Sp 6)   dampness and heat.
Yin Ling Quan (Sp 9)

Chinese medicinal formula: *Huang Qing Hua Shi Tang* (Scutellaria & Talcum Decoction)

Ingredients: Radix Scutellariae Baicalensis (*Huang Qin*), 10g, Talcum (*Hua Shi*), 10g, Fructus Cardamomi (*Bai Dou Kou*), 6g, Pericarpium Arecae Catechu (*Da Fu Pi*), 10g, Sclerotium Polypori Umbellati (*Zhu Ling*), 10g, Cortex Sclerotii Poriae Cocos Poriae (*Fu Ling Pi*), 10g, Herba Agastachis Seu Pogostemi (*Huo Xiang*), 10g, Fructus Xanthii Sibirici (*Cang Er Zi*), 10g

4. Dual vacuity of the lungs & spleen

Symptoms: Diminished sense of smell, nasal congestion accompanied by runny nose with white, sticky nasal mucous, alternately better or worse, cloudedness and distention in the head, shortness of breath, disinclination to speak, fatigue, reduced food intake, abdominal distention, a pale tongue with thin, white fur, and a slow pulse

Therapeutic principles: Warm and supplement the lung qi to dissipate wind cold if the lung qi is vacuous. Nourish yin and moisten dryness if there is dry nose with absence of runny nose. Supplement the center and boost qi when there is spleen vacuity.

Acupuncture & moxibustion:

Ying Xiang (LI 20)   Together, these points harmonize the qi and blood
Ying Tang (M-HN-3)   in the nose to unblock the portals.

Tai Yuan (Lu 9)   Together, these points bank earth and engender
Zu San Li (St 36)   the metal to supplement and boost qi. Select
Pi Shu (Bl 20)   two points each treatment.
Fei Shu (Bl 13)

He Gu (LI 4)   Supplements the qi with supplementing method or resolves the exterior with draining method.

Chinese medicinal formulas:

If lung qi vacuity is predominant: Modified *Wen Fei Zhi Liu Dan* (Warm the Lungs & Stop Flow Elixir)

Ingredients: Radix Panacis Ginseng (*Ren Shen*), 6g, Radix Astragali Membranacei (*Huang Qi*), 15g, Herba Schizonepetae Tenuifoliae (*Jing Jie*), 6g, Herba Cum Radice Asari (*Xi Xin*), 3g, Radix Platycodi Grandiflori (*Jie Geng*), 6g, Fructus Xanthii Sibirici (*Cang Er Zi*), 10g

If spleen qi vacuity is predominant: Modified *Shen Ling Bai Zhu San* (Ginseng, Poria & Actractylodes Powder)

Ingredients: Radix Panacis Ginseng (*Ren Shen*), 6g, Sclerotium Poriae Cocos (*Fu Ling*), 10g, Rhizoma Atractylodis Macrocephalae (*Bai Zhu*), 10g, Radix Dioscoreae Oppositae (*Shan Yao*), 10g, Semen Nelumbinis Nuciferae (*Lian Zi*), 10g, Radix Platycodi Grandiflori (*Jie Geng*), 6g, Fructus Amomi (*Sha Ren*), 6g, Herba Cum Radice Asari (*Xi Xin*), 3g, Fructus Xanthii Sibirici (*Cang Er Zi*), 10g, mix-fried Radix Glycyrrhizae (*Zhi Gan Cao*), 3g

5. Qi stagnation & blood stasis

Symptoms: Diminished or completely lost sense of smell, nasal congestion often present, possible runny nose, cloudedness and oppression in the head, severe headache, cough, a dull tongue with possible static macules, and a fine, choppy pulse

Therapeutic principles: Regulate and harmonize the qi and blood, move stagnation and transform stasis

Acupuncture & moxibustion:

Ying Xiang (LI 20) *Ying Tang* (M-HN-3)	Together, these points move stagnation and dispel stasis to unblock the portals.
He Gu (LI 4) *Feng Chi* (GV 20)	Together, these points course and resolve external evils.
Fei Shu (Bl 13) *Pi Shu* (Bl 20)	Together, these points support the correct and harmonize the qi and blood.

Chinese medicinal formula: Modified *Tong Qiao Huo Xue Tang* (Open the Portals & Quicken the Blood Decoction)

Ingredients: Radix Rubrus Paeoniae Lactiflorae (*Chi Shao*), 10g, Radix Ligustici Wallichii (*Chuan Xiong*), 12g, Radix Angelicae Sinensis (*Dang Gui*), 10g, Flos Carthami Tinctorii (*Hong Hua*), 10g, Radix Platycodi Grandiflori (*Jie Geng*), 6g, Herba Cum Radice Asari (*Xi Xin*), 3g, Rhizoma Acori Graminei (*Shi Chang Pu*), 10g

6. Dual vacuity of the qi & blood

Symptoms: Loss of the sense of smell, free or only slightly inhibited flow of air through the nasal cavity, scant nasal mucous, dizziness, heart palpitations, shortness of breath, lack of strength, a grey tongue with thin fur, and a fine, weak pulse

Therapeutic principles: Supplement the qi and nourish the blood

Acupuncture & moxibustion:

Ying Xiang (LI 20) *Ying Tang* (M-HN-3)	Together, these points quicken the network vessels to unblock the portals.

San Yin Jiao (Sp 6)   Together, these points supplement and boost the
Ge Shu (Bl 17)   qi and blood. Select 2-4 points each treatment.
Fei Shu (Bl 13)
Xin Shu (Bl 15)
Pi Shu (Bl 20)
Zu San Li (St 36)

Chinese medicinal formula: *Ba Zhen Tang* (Eight Pearls Decoction)

Ingredients: Prepared Radix Rehmanniae (*Shu Di*), 12g, Radix Albus Paeoniae Lactiflorae (*Bai Shao*), 10g, Radix Angelicae Sinensis (*Dang Gui*), 10g, Radix Ligustici Wallichii (*Chuan Xiong*), 10g, Radix Codonopsis Pilosulae (*Dang Shen*), 10g, Rhizoma Atractylodis Macrocephalae (*Bai Zhu*), 10g, Sclerotium Poriae Cocos (*Fu Ling*), 10g, mix-fried Radix Glycyrrhizae (*Zhi Gan Cao*), 6g

31
Foul-smelling Nose (Bi Chou)

Foul-smelling nose refers to an offensive odor coming from the nose when breathing. It is mainly encountered in deep-source nasal congestion.

Disease causes, disease mechanisms:

I. Liver/gallbladder damp heat

Damp heat may come from externally contracted dampness and heat which enter the interior or from addiction to fatty and/or sweet foods which ferments dampness and engenders heat. If damp heat goes upward and then congests and brews in the nose, the blood and flesh there will putrefy. Therefore, foul-smelling nasal breath may result.

2. Damp heat from spleen vacuity

Spleen vacuity may result from dietary irregularity, taxation, constitutional vacuity, etc. If there is spleen vacuity, the clear qi cannot be upborne, while turbid yin cannot be downborne. In that case, turbid yin may congest in the nose. With time, this congested turbid yin will transform heat. If damp heat brews and fumes in the nose, the blood and flesh there will putrefy, and, therefore, the breath coming from the nose is offensive.

3. Brewing foulness from visceral disease

In the late stage of wasting thirst disease or yin water pattern, evils will fume and steam the qi and blood and body fluids, engendering foul and turbid qi. When this foul and turbid qi is exhaled through the nose, there will be foul-smelling nasal breath.

Treatment based on pattern discrimination:

I. Liver/gallbladder damp heat

Symptoms: Foul-smelling nasal breath, runny nose with yellow-green nasal mucous, nasal congestion, and a diminished sense of smell. Other symptoms may include headache, local pain in the nostrils when pressed, possible dizziness, red eyes and face, dry mouth and throat, dry stools, dark-colored urine, a red tongue with yellow fur, and a wiry, slippery pulse.

Therapeutic principles: Clear and drain liver/gallbladder damp heat, resolve toxins and unblock the portals

Acupuncture & moxibustion:

Tai Chong (Liv 3)	The source point of the liver channel
Feng Chi (GB 20)	The meeting point of the yang linking vessel Together, these points clear and drain the liver and gallbladder especially when there is a concomitant exterior pattern.
Yin Ling Quan (Sp 9)	Together, these points disinhibit damp heat in the
Qu Quan (Liv 8)	liver/gallbladder.
Shang Xing (GV 23)	Together, these points unblock the network
Ying Xiang (LI 20)	vessels to disinhibit the portals.

Chinese medicinal formula: Modified *Long Dan Xie Gan Tang* (Gentiana Drain the Liver Decoction)

Ingredients: Radix Gentianae Scabrae (*Long Dan Cao*), *6g*, Radix Scutellariae Baicalensis (*Huang Qin*), 10g, Fructus Gardeniae Jasminoidis (*Zhi Zi*), 10g, Rhizoma Alismatis (*Ze Xie*), 6g, uncooked Radix Rehmanniae (*Sheng Di*), 6g, Semen Plantaginis (*Che Qian Zi*), 6g, Flos Lonicerae Japonicae (*Yin Hua*), 15g, Flos Magnoliae Liliflorae (*Xin Yi Hua*), 10g, Herba Cum Radice Taraxaci Mongolici (*Pu Gong Ying*), 10g, Herba Cum Radice Houttuyniae Cordatae (*Yu Xing Cao*), 10g

2. Damp heat from spleen vacuity

Symptoms: Terribly foul-smelling nasal breath, dry, yellow-green scabs inside the nostrils, diminished or absent sense of smell, oppression in the stomach and distention in the abdomen, headache, desire for sleep, lassitude of the spirit, lack of strength, dry mouth with no desire to drink, slimy, white or dry, yellow tongue fur, and a soggy, rapid pulse

Therapeutic principles: Transform dampness and clear heat

Acupuncture and moxibustion:

Shang Xing (GV 23)	Together, these points unblock the network
Ying Xiang (LI 20)	vessels to disinhibit the portals.
Ying Tang (M-HN-3)	
Zhong Wan (CV 12)	The alarm point of the stomach
Gong Sun (Sp 4)	The network point of the spleen
	Together, these points fortify the spleen to transform the dampness when needled with moderate manipulation.
Yin Ling Quan (Sp 9)	The uniting point of the spleen
Feng Long (St 40)	The network point of the stomach
	Together, these points transform phlegm, disinhibit dampness, and clear heat when needled with draining method.

Chinese medicinal formula: Modified *Huang Qin Hua Shi Tang* (Scutellaria & Talcum Decoction)

Ingredients: Radix Scutellariae Baicalensis (*Huang Qin*), 10g, Talcum (*Hua Shi*), 10g, Sclerotium Poriae Cocos (*Fu Ling*), 10g, Sclerotium Polypori Umbellati (*Zhu Ling*), 10g, Pericarpium Arecae Catechu (*Da Fu Pi*), 10g, Fructus Cardamomi (*Bai Dou Kou*), 3g, Fructus Amomi (*Sha Ren*), 6g

3. Brewing foulness from visceral disease

Symptoms: The nasal breath is offensive. In the late stage of wasting thirst disease, the symptoms may include nausea, vomiting, poor appetite, abdominal pain, and fatigue followed by desire for sleep, and deep, rapid breathing which smells like rotten apples. In the late stage of yin water pattern, the symptoms are a bad nose smell like urine, a sallow yellow facial complexion, low back ache, fatigue, lack of strength, no thought of food, oppression in the chest and a burning sensation in the region of the heart.

Therapeutic principles: For wasting thirst disease, enrich yin and supplement the kidneys if there is yin vacuity, and enrich the kidneys and warm yang if there is dual vacuity of yin and yang. For yin water pattern, warm and supplement the spleen and kidneys, transform dampness and downbear turbidity.

Acupuncture & moxibustion: Acupuncture and moxibustion do not work very well for this pattern.

Chinese medicinal formulas:

For wasting thirst disease:

If there is yin vacuity: Modified *Liu Wei Di Huang Wan* (Six Flavors Rehmannia Pills)

Ingredients: Uncooked Radix Rehmanniae (*Sheng Di*), 12g, Fructus Corni Officinalis (*Shan Zhu Yu*), 10g, Radix Dioscoreae Oppositae (*Shan Yao*), 15g, Sclerotium Poriae Cocos (*Fu Ling*), 10g, Rhizoma Alismatis (*Ze Xie*), 6g, Cortex Radicis Moutan (*Dan Pi*), 6g, Radix Astragali Membranacei (*Huang Qi*), 15g, Radix Polygoni Multiflori (*He Shou Wu*), 10g

If there is dual vacuity of yin and yang: Modified *Shen Qi Wan* (Kidney Qi Pills)

Ingredients: Uncooked Radix Rehmanniae (*Sheng Di*), 12g, Fructus Corni Officinalis (*Shan Zhu Yu*), 10g, Radix Dioscoreae Oppositae (*Shan Yao*), 15g, Sclerotium Poriae Cocos (*Fu Ling*), 10g, Rhizoma Alismatis (*Ze Xie*), 6g, Cortex Radicis Moutan (*Dan Pi*), 6g, Radix Astragali Membranacei (*Huang Qi*), 15g, Radix Lateralis Praeparatus Aconiti Carmichaeli (*Fu Zi*), 3g, Cortex Cinnamomi Cassiae (*Rou Gui*), 3g, Herba Epimedii (*Xian Ling Pi*), 10g

For yin water pattern: *Wu Zhu Yu Tang* (Evodia Decoction) plus *Fu Zi Li Zhong Tang* (Aconite Rectify the Center Decoction)

Ingredients: Fructus Evodiae Rutecarpae (*Wu Zhu Yu*), 3g, Radix Codonopsis Pilosulae (*Dang Shen*), 10g, uncooked Rhizoma Zingiberis (*Sheng Jiang*), 3g, Fructus Zizyphi Jujubae (*Da Zao*), 5 fruits, Radix Lateralis Praeparatus Aconiti Carmichaeli (*Fu Zi*), 3g, dry Rhizoma Zingiberis (*Gan Jiang*), 6g, Rhizoma Atractylodis Macrocephalae (*Bai Zhu*), 12g, mix-fried Radix Glycyrrhizae (*Zhi Gan Cao*), 6g

32
Nasal Swelling *(Bi Zhong)*

Nasal swelling refers to redness and swelling of the nostrils, especially the lower nostrils.

Disease causes, disease mechanisms:

I. Heat toxins congesting in the lungs

Heat toxins may arise from externally contracted heat evils which enter the interior and congest in the lungs or from addiction to fatty and/or spicy foods which engenders heat internally. "The lungs open into the portal of the nose" and the stomach channel starts at the sides of the nose. If the heat toxins ascend along the channel and congest in the region of the nose, the flow of qi and blood will become stagnant in the network vessels. Therefore, swelling of the nose may occur.

2. Heat toxins falling inward to the constructive & blood aspects

If heat toxins congesting in the lungs are too strong to be cleared and resolved in time or if the patient repeatedly presses the swelling, thus scattering the heat toxins, they may fall inward into the constructive and blood aspects. Therefore, there is nose swelling accompanied by symptoms from heat toxins falling inward into the constructive and blood.

3. *Gan* heat attacking the lungs

In children, the spleen and stomach are still weak and can be easily damaged. If fed improperly, their spleen may be rendered vacuous at the same time that stagnant food brews in their stomach. If there is spleen vacuity with hot food stagnation, damp heat will be engendered internally. If heat brews internally and ascends along the stomach channel to the nose, this may lead to inhibited flow of qi and blood. Then the heat will congest with the stagnant qi and blood and fume and steam in the local area. Thus swelling of the nose may occur.

4. Depressed damp heat steaming in the nose

Damp heat can be externally contracted or internally engendered from spleen/stomach vacuity. If this damp heat goes upward along the stomach channel and becomes depressed in the nose, it may fume and steam there. Therefore, swelling of the nose may occur.

Treatment based on pattern discrimination:

I. Heat toxins congesting in the lungs

Symptoms: The swelling and pain start with a red, burning miliary sore which has a hard root. A pustule then appears on top of this sore in 3-5 days. When this pustule ruptures, the pus drains and the swelling is dispersed. During its course and especially during its early stage, symptoms such as high fever with aversion to cold, headache, thirst, a red tongue with yellow fur, and a rapid pulse may be seen.

Therapeutic principles: Clear heat, resolve toxins, and disperse swelling

Acupuncture & moxibustion:

Shao Shang (Lu 11)	Together, these points clear heat and resolve
Er Jian (LI 2)	toxins when pricked to bleed.
He Gu (LI 4)	The source point of the stomach channel
Da Zhui (GV 14)	A governing vessel point which governs general yang in the body

Qu Chi (LI 11) The uniting point of the stomach channel which ends at the side of the nose
Together, these points clear heat and diffuse the lungs.

Chinese medicinal formula: Modified *Wu Wei Xiao Du Yin* (Five Flavors Disperse Toxins Drink)

Ingredients: Flos Lonicerae Japonicae (*Yin Hua*), 20g, Herba Cum Radice Violae Yedoensitis (*Zi Hua Di Ding*), 10g, Herba Cum Radice Taraxaci Mongolici (*Pu Gong Ying*), 10g, Flos Chrysanthemi Indici (*Ye Ju Hua*), 10g, Radix Semiaquilegiae (*Tian Kui Zi*), 10g, Herba Cum Radice Houttuyniae Cordatae (*Yu Xing Cao*), 10g, Radix Scutellariae Baicalensis (*Huang Qin*), 10g

2. Heat toxins falling inward to the constructive & blood aspects

Symptoms: In the early stage, the symptoms are the same as described above for heat toxins congesting in the lungs. This is then followed by collapse of the top of the sore and an absence of pus. The root of the sore becomes unclear and the head of the sore turns a dull purple. In severe cases, the swelling can make the nose look like a bottle and may involve the lip, cheek, and eyelid. The pain is severe and other symptoms may include high fever, vexation and agitation, nausea and vomiting, thirst, constipation, possible clouded spirit and delirium, convulsive spasm of the limbs, and opisthotonos. The tongue is crimson red, the tongue fur is often yellow and dry, and the pulse is rapid.

Therapeutic principles: Clear the constructive, cool the blood, and resolve toxins

Acupuncture & moxibustion:

Shi Xuan (M-UE-1) Clears the constructive and resolves toxins

Wei Zhong (Bl 40)   The uniting point of the bladder channel
Qu Ze (Per 3)   The uniting point of the pericardium channel
Together, these points cool the blood when
pricked to bleed.

Chinese medicinal formula: *Qing Ying Tang* (Clear the Constructive Decoction)

Ingredients: Cornu Bubali (*Shui Niu Jiao*), 20g, uncooked Radix Rehmanniae (*Sheng Di*), 15g, Radix Scrophulariae Ningpoensis (*Xuan Shen*), 15g, Folium Bambusae (*Zhu Ye*), 10g, Flos Lonicerae Japonicae (*Yin Hua*), 15g, Fructus Forsythiae Suspensae (*Lian Qiao*), 10g, Rhizoma Coptidis Chinensis (*Huang Lian*), 6g, Radix Salviae Miltiorrhizae (*Dan Shen*), 10g, Tuber Ophiopogonis Japonici (*Mai Dong*), 6g

3. Gan heat attacking the lungs

Symptoms: The nostril is swollen but the pain is not severe. Subsequently there is, in turn, erosion, scabbing, cracking, and bleeding and that makes the healing difficult. Other symptoms may include fever, headache, constipation, a red tongue with yellow fur, and a rapid pulse.

Therapeutic principles: Clear heat and resolve toxins

Acupuncture & moxibustion: Acupuncture and moxibustion do not work very well for this pattern.

Chinese medicinal formula: *Qing Jin San* (Clear Metal Powder)

Ingredients: Fructus Gardeniae Jasminoidis (*Zhi Zi*), 10g, Radix Scutellariae Baicalensis (*Huang Qin*), 10g, Folium Eriobotryae Japonicae (*Pi Pa Ye*), 10g, uncooked Radix Rehmanniae (*Sheng Di*), 10g, Radix Trichosanthis Kirlowii (*Tian Hua Fen*), 10g, Fructus Forsythiae Suspensae (*Lian Qiao*), 10g, Tuber Ophiopogonis Japonici (*Mai Dong*),

10g, Herba Menthae Haplocalycis (*Bo He*), 3g, Radix Scrophulariae Ningpoensis (*Xuan Shen*), 10g, Radix Platycodi Grandiflori (*Jie Geng*), 10g, Radix Glycyrrhizae (*Gan Cao*), 6g

4. Depressed damp heat steaming in the nose

Symptoms: The nostril is red, swollen, and distended. There is erosion with yellow water, itching, and pain. Cracking and bleeding may be seen if a scab has formed where the erosion is. This swelling and erosion can involve the wing of the nose and the lips. Other symptoms may include poor appetite, abdominal distention, loose stools, irascibility, crying and restlessness in children, a red tongue with slimy, yellow fur, and a slippery, rapid pulse.

Therapeutic principles: Clear heat and disinhibit dampness

Acupuncture & moxibustion:

He Gu (LI 4)	Together, these points clear heat in the lungs and
Chi Ze (Lu 5)	stomach when needled with draining method.
Nei Ting (St 44)	

Zhong Wan (CV 12)	Together, these points fortify the spleen and
Zu San Li (St 36)	disinhibit dampness when needled with
Yin Ling Guan (Sp 9)	supplementing method.

Chinese medicinal formula: *Chu Shi Tang* (Eliminate Dampness Decoction)

Ingredients: Talcum (*Hua Shi*), 10g, Semen Plantaginis (*Che Qian Zi*), 10g, Radix Scutellariae Baicalensis (*Huang Qin*), 6g, Rhizoma Coptidis Chinensis (*Huang Lian*), 6g, Caulis Akebiae (*Mu Tong*), 3g, Fructus Forsythiae Suspensae (*Lian Qiao*), 10g, Fructus Citri Aurantii (*Zhi Ke*), 10g, Pericarpium Citri Reticulatae (*Chen Pi*), 10g, Sclerotium Poriae Cocos (*Fu Ling*), 10g

33
Sour Nose *(Bi Suan)*

Sour nose refers to a sour smell in the nose as if smelling vinegar. It mainly occurs in the nasal portal or in the root part of the nose.

Disease causes, disease mechanisms:

I. Wind heat congesting in the lungs

Wind heat can be from externally contracted wind heat or wind cold which enters the interior and transforms into heat over time. If wind heat congests in the lungs, it will lead to the non-diffusion of the lung qi and impaired lung depuration. As a result, the portal of the nose will be inhibited. Therefore, there may develop a sour smell in the nose.

2. Phlegm fire blocking the lungs

If fire evils invade the lungs, they may burn humors into phlegm. When this fire combines with this phlegm and blocks the lungs, the diffusion and downbearing function of the lungs will be impaired, leading to inhibition of the portal of the nose. Thus there may be a sour smell in the nose.

3. Lung vacuity coupled with cold invasion

Lung vacuity is often the result of chronic disease, such as enduring cough which consumes the lung qi, or is the result of insufficient engenderment of the qi. Based on the sayings, "The lungs govern the qi," and "The lungs govern the skin and hair", if there is lung qi vacuity, there may be insecurity of the exterior. In that case, cold evils may take advantage of vacuity to invade the body. If cold evils attack the body, the exterior will be fettered, leading to non-diffusion of the lung qi. As a result, the portal of the nose will be inhibited and a sour smell may be felt in the nose.

4. Qi vacuity of the lungs & spleen

The causes of lung qi vacuity are the same as described above. If there is spleen qi vacuity, the clear qi cannot be upborne and turbid yin will not be downborne. If turbid yin congests and attacks the unhealthy nasal portal resulting from lung qi vacuity, a sour smell may occur in the nose.

Note: Although all four of these patterns may be seen in clinical practice, the second pattern is not seen very often.

Treatment based on pattern discrimination:

I. Wind heat congesting in the lungs

Symptoms: A sour smell and distention in the root of the nose which is exacerbated by wind, pain occurring on pressure, runny nose with thick, yellow nasal mucous, fever, aversion to wind, sore throat, thirst, a red tongue with thin, yellow fur, and a rapid pulse

Therapeutic principles: Course wind and clear heat

Acupuncture & moxibustion:

Ying Tang (M-HN-3) *Ying Xiang* (LI 20)	Together, these points course and disperse wind heat from the nose.
He Gu (LI 4) *Feng Chi* (GB 20)	Together, these points course wind and resolve the exterior.
Chi Ze (Lu 5)	Drains heat from the lungs

Additions & subtractions: If there is a sore throat, prick *Shao Shang* (Lu 11) to induce bleeding.

Chinese medicinal formula: *Yin Qiao San* (Lonicera & Forsythia Powder)

Ingredients: Flos Lonicerae Japonicae (*Yin Hua*), 15g, Fructus Forsythiae Suspensae (*Lian Qiao*), 10g, Herba Menthae Haplocalycis (*Bo He*), 6g, Semen Praeparatus Sojae (*Dan Dou Chi*), 6g, Radix Platycodi Grandiflori (*Jie Geng*), 6g, Herba Schizonepetae Tenuifoliae (*Jing Jie*), 10g, Rhizoma Phragmitis Communis (*Lu Gen*), 10g, Folium Bambusae (*Zhu Ye*), 10g, Fructus Arctii Lappae (*Niu Bang Zi*), 10g, Radix Glycyrrhizae (*Gan Cao*), 3g

2. Phlegm fire blocking the lungs

Symptoms: A painful, sour sensation in the nose, runny nose with sticky, thick nasal mucous, nasal congestion, diminished sense of smell, cough with profuse phlegm, heavy-headedness, headache, sticky, slimy, yellow tongue fur, and a slippery, rapid pulse

Therapeutic principles: Clear heat and transform phlegm

Acupuncture & moxibustion:

Ying Tang (M-HN-3)	Together, these points disinhibit the portal of the
Ying Xiang (LI 20)	nose.

Chi Ze (Lu 5)	Together, these points clear heat and transform
Fei Shu (Bl 13)	phlegm.

Additions & subtractions: For headache, add *Tou Wei* (St 8).

Chinese medicinal formula: Modified *Wen Dan Tang* (Warm the Gallbladder Decoction)

Ingredients: Caulis Bambusae In Taeniis (*Zhu Ru*), 10g, Rhizoma Pinelliae Ternatae (*Ban Xia*), 10g, Fructus Immaturus Citri Aurantii (*Zhi Shi*), 6g, Pericarpium Citri Reticulatae (*Chen Pi*), 6g, Sclerotium Poriae Cocos (*Fu Ling*), 10g, Herba Cum Radice Houttuyniae Cordatae (*Yu Xing Cao*), 10g, Radix Scutellariae Baicalensis (*Huang Qin*), 6g, Flos Magnoliae Liliflorae (*Xin Yi Hua*), 10g, Radix Glycyrrhizae (*Gan Cao*), 3g

3. Lung vacuity coupled with cold invasion

Symptoms: A sour smell in the nose which occurs when exposed to cold, nasal congestion, runny nose with clear nasal mucous, lassitude of the spirit, shortness of breath, a weak cough and asthma, dyspnea on movement, a pale tongue with thin fur, and a fine, weak pulse

Therapeutic principles: Boost the qi and secure the exterior, diffuse the lungs and unblock the portals

Acupuncture & moxibustion:

Ying Xiang (LI 20)	Together, these points unblock the portal of nose.
Ying Tang (M-HN-3)	
Tai Yuan (Lu 9)	Together, these points engender the metal viscus
Gao Huang Shu (Bl 43)	to secure the exterior when needled with
Fei Shu (Bl 13)	supplementing method.

Additions & subtractions: If the exterior pattern is marked, add *He Gu* (LI 4).

Chinese medicinal formula: Modified *Yu Ping Feng San* (Jade Windscreen Powder)

Ingredients: Radix Astragali Membranacei (*Huang Qi*), 15g, Rhizoma Atractylodis Macrocephalae (*Bai Zhu*), 10g, Radix Ledebouriellae

Divaricatae (*Fang Feng*), 10g, Flos Magnoliae Liliflorae (*Xin Yi Hua*), 10g, Herba Cum Radice Asari (*Xi Xin*), 3g

4. Qi vacuity of the lungs & spleen

Symptoms: A sour smell and distention in the root of the nose, nasal congestion, runny nose with typically sticky, white nasal mucous, clouded head with headache, lingering cough, shortness of breath, lack of strength, abdominal distention, loose stools, a pale tongue with white fur, and a fine, weak pulse

Therapeutic principles: Boost the qi, fortify the spleen, and transform dampness

Acupuncture & moxibustion:

Ying Xiang (LI 20)	Together, these points unblock and disinhibit the
Ying Tang (M-HN-3)	portal of the nose.
Fei Shu (Bl 13)	The back transporting point of the lungs
Pi Shu (Bl 20)	The back transporting point of the spleen
	Together, these points boost the qi and fortify the
	spleen to transform dampness.
Shan Zhong (CV 17)	The meeting point of the qi
Zu San Li (St 36)	The uniting point of the stomach channel
	Together, these points boost the qi.

Chinese medicinal formula: Modified *Si Jun Zi Tang* (Four Gentlemen Decoction)

Ingredients: Radix Panacis Ginseng (*Ren Shen*), 6g, Rhizoma Atractylodis Macrocephalae (*Bai Zhu*), 10g, Sclerotium Poriae Cocos (*Fu Ling*), 10g, Radix Astragali Membranacei (*Huang Qi*), 15g, mix-fried Radix Glycyrrhizae (*Zhi Gan Cao*), 6g, Flos Magnoliae Liliflorae (*Xin Yi Hua*), 10g

34
Cold Nose *(Bi Leng)*

Cold nose refers to a lack of warmth in the skin of the nose or to cold breath issuing from the nose.

Disease causes, disease mechanisms:

Spleen yang vacuity

Spleen yang vacuity may develop from dietary irregularity, such as addiction to cold and raw food, or from overdosage and/or enduring administration of cold, cool medicinals which damage spleen yang. Yang is responsible for warming the body. Therefore, if there is spleen yang vacuity, there may be a chilly nose.

Treatment based on pattern discrimination:

Spleen yang vacuity

Symptoms: Cold nose, reduced food intake, abdominal distention, cold and pain in the abdomen which is relieved by warmth and pressure, lack of warmth in the limbs, loose stools, a pale tongue with thin fur, and a fine, weak pulse

Therapeutic principles: Warm and supplement spleen yang

Acupuncture & moxibustion:

Bai Hui (GV 20)   Warms yang with moxibustion

Ying Xiang (LI 20)   Helps free the flow of yang in the nose

Guan Yuan (CV 4)   Together, these points warm and supplement
Qi Hai (CV 6)   spleen yang with moxibustion.
Zhong Wan (CV 12)

Chinese medicinal formula: Modified *Li Zhong Tang* (Rectify the Center Pills)

Ingredients: Radix Codonopsis Pilosulae (*Dang Shen*), 10g, Rhizoma Atractylodis Macrocephalae (*Bai Zhu*), 10g, dry Rhizoma Zingiberis (*Gan Jiang*), 6g, Herba Cum Radice Asari (*Xi Xin*), 3g, mix-fried Radix Glycyrrhizae (*Zhi Gan Cao*), 6g

Note: The development of a cold nose when seen in a life-threatening disease is a sign of immanent death.

35
Sore, Swollen Throat *(Yan Hou Zhong Tong)*

This refers to painful swelling and distention on one or both sides of the throat. In some cases, the whole throat may be involved and uvular ptosis can be seen when involved.

Disease causes, disease mechanisms:

I. Wind heat invasion

When wind heat invades the body, it often does so by way of the mouth and nose. The throat is where the nose and mouth meet. If wind heat congests in the throat, it will cause stagnation of the qi and blood there. Thus there may be a sore, swollen throat. If wind heat enters the lungs and congests there, heat may become even more exuberant, leading to an even more severe sore, swollen throat if this heat ascends and burns the throat.

2. Exuberant heat of the lungs & stomach coupled with wind invasion

Lung heat exuberance is often the result of externally contracted wind heat or wind cold that has not been dispelled. This then enters and congests in the lungs. Stomach heat exuberance mainly arises from addiction to alcohol or spicy and/or fatty foods which brews and engenders heat. The pharynx connects with the stomach and the larynx to the lungs. If exuberant heat is stirred by an external contraction of wind, it will go upward, congesting and burning in the throat. Hence the flow of qi and blood may be inhibited and this may produce soreness and swelling in the throat.

3. Lung yin vacuity

Lung yin vacuity may develop from heat evils and/or dry evils that damage the liquids or from chronic lung disease that consumes the liquids of the lungs. When there is lung yin vacuity, first, the throat will not be moistened sufficiently and, secondly, yin vacuity fire may go upward and burn the throat. Therefore, sore swollen throat occurs.

4. Kidney yin vacuity

Kidney yin vacuity may be due to congenital insufficiency, sexual taxation, chronic disease, or aging. If there is kidney yin vacuity, the throat will not be sufficiently nourished. In addition, yin vacuity fire may ascend, congesting in and burning the throat. Therefore, sore swollen throat results.

Treatment based on pattern discrimination:

I. Wind heat invasion

Symptoms: In the early stage, one or both sides of the throat are dry, red, and swollen with slight burning pain. There may also be some small, red spots like sudamina found on the mucous membranes. This redness and swelling may get worse and be accompanied by fever, sweating, headache, cough, etc. The tongue is red with thin, yellow fur, and the pulse is typically floating and rapid.

Therapeutic principles: Course wind and clear heat

Acupuncture & moxibustion:

Feng Men (Bl 12)   Wind points; together, they course wind.
Feng Chi (GB 20)

Chi Ze (Lu 5)   Together, these points diffuse the lungs and clear
Qu Chi (LI 11)   heat.

Tian Tu (CV 22)	Together, these points resolve the exterior and
Wai Guan (TB 5)	clear heat, disinhibit the throat and transform phlegm.

Chinese medicinal formula: Modified *Yin Qiao San* (Lonicera & Forsythia Powder)

Ingredients: Flos Lonicerae Japonicae (*Yin Hua*), 15g, Fructus Forsythiae Suspensae (*Lian Qiao*), 10g, Herba Menthae Haplocalycis (*Bo He*), 6g, Radix Platycodi Grandiflori (*Jie Geng*), 12g, Herba Schizonepetae Tenuifoliae (*Jing Jie*), 10g, Folium Bambusae (*Zhu Ye*), 10g, Fructus Arctii Lappae (*Niu Bang Zi*), 12g, Periostracum Cicadae (*Chan Tui*), 10g, Radix Scrophulariae Ningpoensis (*Xuan Shen*), 10g

2. Exuberant heat of the lungs & stomach coupled with wind invasion

Symptoms: The throat is red, swollen, and severely painful. There is a blocked sensation when swallowing and, in severe cases, the pain extends to the ear, thus making swallowing even more difficult. Other symptoms include cough with profuse, sticky, thick phlegm, possible nodules in the neck which hurt on pressure, alternating chills and fever or persistent high fever, thirst with desire to drink, dry stools and constipation, a red tongue with yellow fur, and a surging, rapid pulse.

Therapeutic principles: Course wind and clear the heat, resolve toxins and disinhibit the throat

Acupuncture & moxibustion:

Shao Shang (Lu 11)	Together, these points clear heat and drain fire to
Shang Yang (LI 1)	disperse the swelling and stop the pain when
Li Dui (St 45)	pricked to let 3-5 drops of blood.

Lian Quan (CV 23)	Clears heat and disinhibits the throat

San Jian (LI 3)	Frees the stool to drain heat based on the saying,
Tian Shu (St 25)	"Withdraw the firewood from under the pot."
Feng Long (St 40)	

Chinese medicinal formula: Modified *Qing Yan Li Ge Tang* (Clear the Throat & Disinhibit the Diaphragm Decoction)

Ingredients: Radix Scutellariae Baicalensis (*Huang Qin*), 10g, Herba Menthae Haplocalycis (*Bo He*), 6g, Fructus Forsythiae Suspensae (*Lian Qiao*), 10g, Fructus Gardeniae Jasminoidis (*Zhi Zi*), 6g, Fructus Arctii Lappae (*Niu Bang Zi*), 12g, Rhizoma Cimicifugae (*Sheng Ma*), 10g, Radix Platycodi Grandiflori (*Jie Geng*), 10g, Flos Lonicerae Japonicae (*Yin Hua*),10g, Radix Scrophulariae Ningpoensis (*Xuan Shen*), 10g, Rhizoma Coptidis Chinensis (*Huang Lian*), 6g, Mirabilitum (*Mang Xiao*), 6g, Radix Et Rhizoma Rhei (*Da Huang*), 6g, Radix Glycyrrhizae (*Gan Cao*), 9g

3. Lung yin vacuity

Symptoms: Only discomfort or slight pain in the throat, slight redness and swelling of the throat. The patient often tries to relieve this uncomfortable sensation as if there were a foreign body in the throat by coughing. There is also a dry throat and tongue, red cheeks and lips, heat in the palms of the hands and soles of the feet, and lassitude of the spirit. Usually, the symptoms are minor in the morning, mild in the afternoon, and severe at night. Other symptoms are a dry cough, a bright red tongue with no fur, and a fine, rapid or floating, fine pulse.

Therapeutic principles: Nourish yin and clear the lungs

Acupuncture & moxibustion:

Lian Quan (CV 23)	Disinhibits and moistens the throat
Lie Que (Lu 7)	Together, these points enrich lung and kidney yin
Zhao Hai (Ki 6)	to clear and downbear the floating ministerial fire.

Tai Xi (Ki 3)	Together, these points enrich and supplement yin
San Yin Jiao (Sp 6)	to check exuberant yang.
Yu Ji (Lu 10)	Diffuses the lungs and clears heat to disinhibit the throat

Chinese medicinal formula: *Yang Yin Qing Fei Tang* (Nourish Yin & Clear the Lungs Decoction)

Ingredients: Uncooked Radix Rehmanniae (*Sheng Di*), 10g, Tuber Ophiopogonis Japonici (*Mai Dong*), 10g, Radix Scrophulariae Ningpoensis (*Xuan Shen*), 10g, Bulbus Fritillariae Cirrhosae (*Chuan Bei Mu*), 6g, Cortex Radicis Moutan (*Dan Pi*), 6g, Herba Menthae Haplocalycis (*Bo He*), 6g, Radix Albus Paeoniae Lactiflorae (*Bai Shao*), 6g, Radix Glycyrrhizae (*Gan Cao*), 6g

4. Kidney yin vacuity

Symptoms: The main symptoms are the same as those for lung yin vacuity, however, with the addition to specifically kidney vacuity signs and symptoms, such as low back and knee pain and weakness, tinnitus, flowery, (*i.e.*, blurred vision), vacuity vexation and insomnia, a red tongue with scant fur, and a fine, rapid pulse.

Therapeutic principles: Enrich yin and downbear fire

Acupuncture and moxibustion: Use the same prescription as for lung yin vacuity but subtract *Yu Ji* (Lu 10) while adding *Shen Shu* (Bl 23).

Chinese medicinal formula: Modified *Zhi Bai Di Huang Wan* (Anemarrhena & Phellodendron Rehmannia Pills)

Ingredients: Rhizoma Anemarrhenae Asphodeloidis (*Zhi Mu*), 10g, Cortex Phellodendri (*Huang Bai*), 10g, Radix Scrophulariae Ningpoensis (*Xuan Shen*), 12g, uncooked Radix Rehmanniae (*Sheng Di*), 12g, Fructus

Corni Officinalis (*Shan Zhu Yu*), 10g, Radix Dioscoreae Oppositae (*Shan Yao*), 6g, Rhizoma Alismatis (*Ze Xie*), 6g, Tuber Ophiopogonis Japonici (*Mai Dong*), 10g, Sclerotium Poriae Cocos (*Fu Ling*), 6g, Cortex Cinnamomi Cassiae (*Rou Gui*), 1g

36
Baby Moth Swollen Tonsil *(Hou Qi Zhong Kuai)*

Baby moth swollen tonsil refers to redness and enlargement of one or both tonsils. It is called this because the tonsils, when inflamed and purulent, look like a baby moth.

Disease causes, disease mechanisms:

The disease causes and disease mechanisms for baby moth swollen tonsil are essentially the same as for sore, swollen throat discussed above.

Treatment based on pattern discrimination:

I. Wind heat invading the throat

Symptoms: Pain in the throat which gets worse gradually and is exacerbated by swallowing and coughing, a dry throat with a burning sensation, red, swollen tonsils and throat, fever with aversion to cold, headache, nasal congestion, fatigue, cough with phlegm, a red tongue tip and edges with thin, white or thin, yellow fur, and a floating, rapid pulse

Therapeutic principles: Course wind and clear heat, disperse swelling and disinhibit the throat

Acupuncture and moxibustion:

Shao Shang (Lu 11)   The well point of the lungs; clears heat in the lungs and disinhibits the throat when pricked to let 5-15 drops of blood.

He Gu (LI 4)	The source point of the large intestine channel; courses wind and clears heat.
Qu Chi (LI 11)	The uniting point of the large intestine channel; clears heat in combination with *He Gu*.
Tian Rong (SI 17)	An empirically effective point for baby moth; clears heat, disperses swelling, and disinhibits the throat.

Remarks: The above is a simple but effective prescription. Draining method should be used on all the points not bled.

Chinese medicinal formula: Modified *Yin Qiao San* (Lonicera & Forsythia Powder)

Ingredients: Flos Lonicerae Japonicae (*Yin Hua*), 15g, Fructus Forsythiae Suspensae (*Lian Qiao*), 10g, Herba Menthae Haplocalycis (*Bo He*), 6g, Radix Platycodi Grandiflori (*Jie Geng*), 12g, Herba Schizonepetae Tenuifoliae (*Jing Jie*), 10g, Folium Bambusae (*Zhu Ye*), 10g, Fructus Arctii Lappae (*Niu Bang Zi*), 12g, Periostracum Cicadae (*Chan Tui*), 10g, Radix Scrophulariae Ningpoensis (*Xuan Shen*), 10g

2. Exuberant heat of the lungs & stomach coupled with wind invasion

Symptoms: Severe throat pain extending to the retroauricular, subauricular, and submaxillary regions, difficulty swallowing, a blocked sensation, hoarse voice, red, swollen tonsil(s) with possible white spots which connect to make a false membrane covering the tonsil(s), in severe cases, redness and swelling of the isthmus of the fauces, palpable submaxillary nodes which are painful on pressure. Other symptoms may include high fever, thirst with desire to drink, cough with thick, yellow phlegm, bad breath, abdominal distention, constipation, dark-colored urine, a red tongue with thick, yellow fur, and a surging, large, rapid pulse.

Therapeutic principles: Drain heat and resolve toxins, disinhibit the throat and disperse swelling

Acupuncture & moxibustion: Use the same prescription as for wind heat invasion above but add in *Nei Ting* (St 44) in combination with *Qu Chi* so as to enhance its action of draining stomach fire.

Chinese medicinal formula: Modified *Qing Yan Li Ge Tang* (Clear the Throat & Disinhibit Diaphragm Decoction)

Ingredients: Radix Scutellariae Baicalensis (*Huang Qin*), 10g, Herba Menthae Haplocalycis (*Bo He*), 6g, Fructus Forsythiae Suspensae (*Lian Qiao*), 10g, Fructus Gardeniae Jasminoidis (*Zhi Zi*), 6g, Fructus Arctii Lappae (*Niu Bang Zi*), 12g, Rhizoma Cimicifugae (*Sheng Ma*), 10g, Radix Platycodi Grandiflori (*Jie Geng*), 10g, Flos Lonicerae Japonicae (*Yin Hua*), 10g, Radix Scrophulariae Ningpoensis (*Xuan Shen*), 10g, Rhizoma Coptidis Chinensis (*Huang Lian*), 6g, Mirabilitum (*Mang Xiao*), 6g, Radix Et Rhizoma Rhei (*Da Huang*), 6g, Radix Glycyrrhizae (*Gan Cao*), 9g

3. Lung yin vacuity

Symptoms: Dry, burning discomfort in the throat accompanied by slight pain and itching which the patient often tries to relieve by deliberate coughing, enlarged tonsils with possible yellowish white pus spots on them, worsening of symptoms in the afternoon. Other symptoms may include afternoon red checks, dry cough with no or scant, sticky phlegm, lassitude of the spirit, heat in the palms of the hands and soles of the feet, a low voice, a red tongue with possible dry, scant fur, and a fine, rapid pulse.

Therapeutic principles: Nourish yin and clear the lungs, engender liquids and moisten dryness

Acupuncture & moxibustion:

Tian Rong (SI 17) *Yu Ji* (Lu 10) *He Gu* (LI 4)	Together, these points clear heat from the lungs and disinhibit the throat.
Lie Que (Lu 7) *Zhao Hai* (Ki 6)	Together, these points nourish yin to downbear fire.

Chinese medicinal formula: *Yang Yin Qing Fei Tang* (Nourish Yin & Clear the Lungs Decoction)

Ingredients: Uncooked Radix Rehmanniae (*Sheng Di*), 10g, Tuber Ophiopogonis Japonici (*Mai Dong*), 10g, Radix Scrophulariae Ningpoensis (*Xuan Shen*), 10g, Bulbus Fritillariae Cirrhosae (*Chuan Bei Mu*), 6g, Cortex Radicis Moutan (*Dan Pi*), 6g, Herba Menthae Haplocalycis (*Bo He*), 6g, Radix Albus Paeoniae Lactiflorae (*Bai Shao*), 6g, Radix Glycyrrhizae (*Gan Cao*), 6g

4. Kidney yin vacuity

Symptoms: Dry, burning discomfort in the throat which the patient often tries to relieve by deliberate coughing, tidal flushing of the tonsils and surrounding area, possible yellowish white pus spots on the tonsils, white pussy matter discharged from the tonsil when pressed. Other symptoms may include a dry mouth with no desire for profuse drinking, dizziness, flowery, (*i.e.*, blurred), vision, tinnitus, deafness, low back and knee pain and weakness, vacuity vexation and insomnia, a red tongue with scant fur, and a fine, rapid pulse.

Therapeutic principles: Enrich yin and downbear fire

Acupuncture & moxibustion:

Yi Feng (TB 17)   Clears heat from the triple burner, disperses
                         swelling, disinhibits the throat, and stops pain

Tong Li (Ht 5)   Together, these points nourish kidney yin and
San Yin Jiao (Sp 6)   downbear fire.

Chinese medicinal formula: Modified *Zhi Bai Di Huang Wan* (Anemarrhena & Phellodendron Rehmannia Pills)

Ingredients: Rhizoma Anemarrhenae Asphodeloidis (*Zhi Mu*), 10g, Cortex Phellodendri (*Huang Bai*), 10g, Radix Scrophulariae Ningpoensis (*Xuan Shen*), 12g, uncooked Radix Rehmanniae (*Sheng Di*), 12g, Fructus Corni Officinalis (*Shan Zhu Yu*), 10g, Radix Dioscoreae Oppositae (*Shan Yao*), 6g, Rhizoma Alismatis (*Ze Xie*), 6g, Tuber Ophiopogonis Japonici (*Mai Dong*), 10g, Sclerotium Poriae Cocos (*Fu Ling*), 6g, Cortex Cinnamomi Cassiae (*Rou Gui*), 1g

37
Itchy Throat *(Yan Yang)*

Itchy throat refers to an uneasy sensation in the throat which calls for relief by scratching with the tongue. This condition usually occurs together with cough, a dry throat, and a hoarse voice. Therefore, the reader should also refer for diagnosis and treatment to each of these other pathoconditions discussed herein.

Disease causes, disease mechanisms:

I. Contraction of external evils

External evils here mainly refer to wind, heat, and dryness. Commonly, heat and dryness combine with wind to invade the body. Wind is a yang evil and its nature is to move. When other external evils invade the body in combination with wind, they fetter the exterior and lead to non-diffusion of the lung qi. Or they may lead to impairment of the lungs' depuration. However, in this case, instead of coming and going through the skin, these external evils come and go through the interstices of the throat which pertains to the lungs. It is this in and out movement of evil qi which often creates itching in the throat.

2. Lung yin vacuity

Lung yin vacuity often arises from chronic disease which consumes yin or heat evils that linger in the lungs. It may also be due to over-sweating due to malpractice, leading to damage of lung yin. The throat pertains to the lungs. If there is lung yin vacuity, the throat may not be sufficiently nourished, and, moreover, yin vacuity fire may flame upward. If this fire is effulgent, pain in the larynx will occur. If this fire is weak, itching will occur instead.

3. Stomach fire fuming & steaming

Stomach fire usually comes from addiction to alcohol or spicy and/or fatty foods which engender heat. If this heat goes upward, fuming and steaming in the throat and itching in the larynx will occur as long as this fire is not very exuberant.

Treatment based on pattern discrimination:

I. Wind heat

Symptoms: Dry, itchy throat which the patient tries to relieve by deliberate coughing, inhibited voice, possible sore throat, fever, sweating, aversion to wind, headache, marked reddening of the mucous membranes in the throat, a red tongue with thin, yellow fur, and a floating, rapid pulse

Therapeutic principles: Course wind and clear heat

Acupuncture & moxibustion:

Shao Shang (Lu 11)   Clears heat when pricked to induce bleeding

He Gu (LI 4)   Together, these points course wind to relieve the
Feng Chi (GB 20)   itching when needled with draining method.

Qu Chi (LI 11)   Together, these points clear heat when needled
Chi Ze (Lu 5)   with draining method.

Chinese medicinal formula: Modified *Sang Ju Yin* (Morus & Chrysanthemum Drink)

Ingredients: Folium Mori Albi (*Sang Ye*), 12g, Flos Chrysanthemi Morifolii (*Ju Hua*), 15g, Herba Menthae Haplocalycis (*Bo He*), 6g, Semen Pruni Armeniacae (*Xing Ren*), 10g, Fructus Forsythiae Suspensae (*Lian Qiao*), 10g, Radix Platycodi Grandiflori (*Jie Geng*), 10g, Rhizoma Phragmitis Communis (*Lu Gen*), 10g, Periostracum Cicadae (*Chan Tui*), 12g, Radix Glycyrrhizae (*Gan Cao*), 10g

2. Wind cold

Symptoms: Itchy throat, cough with clear, thin phlegm, possible slight pain in the throat, inhibited voice, nasal congestion, a heavy voice, runny nose with clear mucous, sneezing, fever, aversion to cold, headache, pale red mucous membranes in the throat, thin, white tongue fur, and a floating, tight pulse

Therapeutic principles: Course wind and scatter cold

Acupuncture & moxibustion:

Lie Que (Lu 7) *Feng Chi* (GB 20)	Together, these points course wind to stop itching when needled with draining method.
He Gu (LI 4) *Wai Guan* (TB 5)	Together, these points course wind and scatter cold when needled with draining method.

Chinese medicinal formula: Modified *Liu Wei Tang* (Six Flavors Decoction)

Ingredients: Radix Ledebouriellae Divaricatae (*Fang Feng*), 10g, Herba Schizonepetae Tenuifoliae (*Jing Jie*), 10g, Herba Menthae Haplocalycis (*Bo He*), 6g, Bombyx Batryticatus (*Jiang Can*), 10g, Radix Platycodi Grandiflori (*Jie Geng*), 10g, Radix Glycyrrhizae (*Gan Cao*), 10g, Periostracum Cicadae (*Chan Tui*), 10g

3. Lung dryness

Symptoms: Itchy throat, dry cough with scant or sticky phlegm which is difficult to expectorate, a dry nose and pharynx, dry tongue with scant liquids, in some cases, sore throat accompanied by cough with blood-streaked phlegm. Other symptoms may include fever with aversion to wind or cold, thin, yellow or thin, white tongue fur, and a floating, rapid or floating, tight pulse.

Therapeutic principles: Diffuse the lungs and moisten dryness

Acupuncture & moxibustion:

He Gu (LI 4)	A combination of source and network points
Lie Que (Lu 7)	associated with the exterior and interior respectively; together, they diffuse the lungs and eliminate evils to stop itching.
Fei Shu (Bl 13)	Moistens dryness of the lungs

Additions & subtractions: Add *Qu Chi* (LI 11) to clear the heat and *San Yin Jiao* (Sp 6) to nourish yin when there are accompanying heat evils. Add *Feng Chi* (GB 20) and *Feng Men* (Bl 12) to course the wind and clear dryness when there are accompanying cold evils.

Chinese medicinal formula: *Sang Xing Tang* (Morus & Armeniaca Decoction)

Ingredients: Folium Mori Albi (*Sang Ye*), 10g, Semen Pruni Armeniacae (*Xing Ren*), 10g, Radix Glehniae Littoralis (*Bei Sha Shen*), 12g, Bulbus Fritillariae Cirrhosae (*Chuan Bei Mu*), 6g, Semen Praeparatus Sojae (*Dan Dou Chi*), 6g, Fructus Gardeniae Jasminoidis (*Zhi Zi*), 10g, Pericarpium Pyri (*Li Pi*), 6g

Additions & subtractions: If there is warm dryness, add Tuber Ophiopogonis Japonici (*Mai Dong*), 10g, and Rhizoma Phragmitis Communis (*Lu Gen*), 10g. If there is cool dryness, add Herba Schizonepetae Tenuifoliae (*Jing Jie*), 10g, and Radix Ledebouriellae Divaricatae (*Fang Feng*), 10g, and subtract Radix Glehniae Littoralis (*Bei Sha Shen*), and Pericarpium Pyri (*Li Pi*).

4. Lung yin vacuity

Symptoms: Minor itchy throat, dry cough with scant or thick phlegm, tidal flushing of the face which is worse in the afternoon, low-grade fever, sweating, thirst but desire for only scant drinking, shortness of breath, disinclination to speak, possible hoarse voice, a red tongue with scant fur, and a fine, rapid pulse

Therapeutic principles: Nourish yin and clear heat

Acupuncture & moxibustion:

Lie Que (Lu 7) *Zhao Hai* (Ki 6)	Together, these points nourish yin and clear heat, moisten the throat and stop itching.
Fei Shu (Bl 13) *Zhong Fu* (Lu 1)	A combination of transporting and alarm points; together, they nourish lung yin.
San Yin Jiao (Sp 6)	A point on the spleen channel; it nourishes yin to enrich lung yin since earth engenders metal.

Chinese medicinal formula: *Bai He Gu Jin Tang* (Lily Secure Metal Decoction)

Ingredients: Bulbus Lilii (*Bai He*), 10g, uncooked Radix Rehmanniae (*Sheng Di*), 10g, prepared Radix Rehmanniae (*Shu Di*), 12g, Tuber Ophiopogonis Japonici (*Mai Dong*), 10g, Rhizoma Anemarrhenae Asphodeloidis (*Zhi Mu*), 10g, Radix Scrophulariae Ningpoensis (*Xuan Shen*), 10g, Radix Platycodi Grandiflori (*Jie Geng*), 6g, Radix Angelicae

Sinensis (*Dang Gui*), 3g, Radix Albus Paeoniae Lactiflorae (*Bai Shao*), 3g, Radix Glycyrrhizae (*Gan Cao*), 6g

5. Stomach fire fuming & steaming

Symptoms: Itchy throat more marked than pain, dry throat, a pale red, slightly swollen throat followed by the gradual appearance of a strawberry-like ulcer. Other symptoms may include thirst, bad breath, dry stools, dark-colored urine, a red tongue, and a rapid or slippery, rapid pulse.

Therapeutic principles: Enrich yin and clear heat

Acupuncture & moxibustion:

Fu Tu (LI 18)	A combination of upper and lower points;
Nei Ting (St 44)	together, they clear heat.
Tian Shu (St 25)	Together, these points free the stools to drain
Shang Ju Xu (St 37)	heat.
San Yin Jiao (Sp 6)	Enriches yin

Chinese medicinal formula: Modified *Qing Wei Tang* (Clear Stomach Decoction)

Ingredients: Uncooked Radix Rehmanniae (*Sheng Di*), 15g, Rhizoma Coptidis Chinensis (*Huang Lian*), 6g, Cortex Radicis Moutan (*Dan Pi*), 6g, Rhizoma Cimicifugae (*Sheng Ma*), 10g, Tuber Ophiopogonis Japonici (*Mai Dong*), 10g, Radix Glehniae Littoralis (*Bei Sha Shen*), 10g

38
Dry Throat *(Yan Gan)*

This refers to a feeling of lacking sufficient moisture in the throat.

Disease causes, disease mechanisms:

I. Wind heat invading the lungs

Wind heat is usually from externally contracted wind heat or from wind cold which enters the interior and transforms into heat. This heat may congest in the lungs and then ascend to fume and steam the throat, thus evaporating the liquids in the throat. Therefore, dry throat may occur.

2. Dry heat damaging the lungs

Dry heat is mainly externally contracted. It is said that, "The lungs are a tender viscus and like moisture, while they dislike dryness." It is also said, "Dry evils damage liquids." Therefore, heat evils may consume yin fluids. If dry heat invades the lungs, first, they will directly damage liquids. Secondly, they will impair the fluid-distributing function of the lungs. Therefore, the throat will be deprived of sufficient moisture and dry throat may occur.

3. Exuberant heat of the spleen & stomach

Exuberant heat may arise from addiction to alcohol and spicy and/or fatty foods which engender heat or from externally contracted evils which enter the interior and transform into heat. Both the spleen channel and the stomach channel connect with the throat. In addition, the pharynx connects with the stomach. If heat goes upward along these channels to the pharynx and steams there, fluids there will be damaged. Therefore, there is a dry throat.

4. Depressive heat in the liver/gallbladder

Depressive heat mainly comes from emotional disturbance, such as anger and frustration, which causes liver depression/qi stagnation. If liver depression/qi stagnation transforms into fire over time, this fire may ascend and steam the throat. Therefore, a dry throat may occur.

5. Lung yin vacuity

Lung yin vacuity may be due to chronic disease which consumes yin or to lingering heat evils in the lungs after a febrile disease. The lungs are responsible for the distribution of yin fluids. If there is lung yin vacuity, there will be less fluids to be distributed in order to moisten the throat. Thus, a dry throat may occur.

6. Kidney yin vacuity

Kidney yin vacuity may be the result of chronic disease, sexual intemperance, aging, etc. If there is kidney yin vacuity, yang will not be checked properly and the frenetic movement of ministerial fire may ensue. If this fire flames upward and burns the throat, fluids there will be damaged and thus a dry throat may occur.

Treatment based on pattern discrimination:

1. Wind heat invading the lungs

Symptoms: Dry throat is often accompanied by painful itching and a burning sensation. There is thirst with desire to drink. Other symptoms may include cough with yellow phlegm, fever, aversion to wind, nasal congestion, a red tongue with thin, white or thin, yellow fur, and a floating, rapid pulse.

Therapeutic principles: Clear heat and diffuse the lungs

Acupuncture & moxibustion:

Lian Quan (CV 23)	Engenders liquid to moisten the throat
Chi Ze (Lu 5) *Fei Shu* (Bl 13)	Together, these points clear heat and protect liquids.
He Gu (LI 4) *Feng Fu* (GV 16)	Together, these points diffuse the lungs and resolve the exterior.

Chinese medicinal formula: *Sang Ju Yin* (Morus & Chrysanthemum Decoction)

Ingredients: Folium Mori Albi (*Sang Ye*), 10g, Flos Chrysanthemi Morifolii (*Ju Hua*), 10g, Semen Pruni Armeniacae (*Xing Ren*), 10g, Herba Menthae Haplocalycis (*Bo He*), 6g, Fructus Forsythiae Suspensae (*Lian Qiao*), 10g, Radix Platycodi Grandiflori (*Jie Geng*), 10g, Radix Glycyrrhizae (*Gan Cao*), 6g, Rhizoma Phragmitis Communis (*Lu Gen*), 10g

2. Dry heat damaging the lungs

Symptoms: A dry throat often accompanied by a dry nose, red mucous membranes in the throat, dry cough with no or scant, sticky phlegm which is difficult to expectorate, chest pain, fever, headache, body aches, a red tongue with thin, white fur, and a floating, fine, rapid pulse

Therapeutic principles: Clear dryness and moisten the lungs

Acupuncture & moxibustion:

Lie Que (Lu 7) *Chi Ze* (Lu 5) *Fei Shu* (Bl 13)	Together, these points clear dry heat and moisten the lungs.

San Yin Jiao (Sp 6) Nourishes yin to help *Fei Shu* moisten the lungs

Additions & subtractions: If there is sore throat, add *Shao Shang* (Lu 11).

Chinese medicinal formula: *Qing Zao Jiu Fei Tang* (Clear Dryness & Rescue the Lungs Decoction)

Ingredients: Folium Mori Albi (*Sang Ye*), 10g, Gypsum Fibrosum (*Shi Gao*), 20g, Radix Codonopsitis Pilosulae (*Dang Shen*), 10g, black Semen Sesami Indici (*Hei Zhi Ma*), 6g, Gelatinum Corii Asini (*E Jiao*), 5g, Tuber Ophiopogonis Japonici (*Mai Dong*), 10g, Semen Pruni Armeniacae (*Xing Ren*), 10g, Folium Eriobotryae Japonicae (*Pi Pa Ye*), 10g, Radix Glycyrrhizae (*Gan Cao*), 6g

3. Exuberant heat of the spleen & stomach

Symptoms: A dry throat often accompanied by dry mouth, vexatious thirst with desire to drink, bad breath, red mucous membranes always present on inspection. Other symptoms may include painful, burning heat in the stomach, acid regurgitation, clamoring stomach, dry stools, dark-colored urine, a red tongue with yellow fur, and a slippery, rapid pulse.

Therapeutic principles: Clear and drain fire from the spleen and stomach

Acupuncture & moxibustion:

Ren Ying (St 9) This point clears fire and protects liquids when tapped with a plum blossom needle.

He Gu (LI 4) Drains heat from the *yang ming*

Zhong Wan (CV 12) Together, these points drain spleen/stomach fire.
Jie Xi (St 41)

San Yin Jiao (Sp 6)   Nourishes and protects stomach yin

Chinese medicinal formula: Modified *Qing Wei San* (Clear Stomach Powder)

Ingredients: Rhizoma Coptidis Chinensis (*Huang Lian*), 6g, uncooked Radix Rehmanniae (*Sheng Di*), 10g, Cortex Radicis Moutan (*Dan Pi*), 6g, Rhizoma Cimicifugae (*Sheng Ma*), 10g, Tuber Ophiopogonis Japonici (*Mai Dong*), 10g, Radix Scrophulariae Ningpoensis (*Xuan Shen*), 10g, Herba Dendrobii (*Shi Hu*), 10g

4. Depressive heat in the liver/gallbladder

Symptoms: A dry throat often accompanied by a bitter taste in the mouth, red mucous membranes in the throat, vertigo, fullness and oppression in the chest and lateral costal regions, vexation, inclination to vomit, a red tongue with thin, yellow fur, and a wiry, fine pulse

Therapeutic principles: Clear the liver and drain the gallbladder

Acupuncture & moxibustion:

Lian Quan (CV 23)   Engenders liquids

Qi Men (Liv 14)   Alarm points; together, they clear heat in the liver
Ri Yue (GB 24)   and gallbladder.

Zhi Gou (TB 6)   Together, these points move the qi and open
Tai Chong (Liv 3)   oppression to help clear heat.

Chinese medicinal formula: *Xie Qing Wan* (Drain the Green Pills)

Ingredients: Radix Gentianae Scabrae (*Long Dan Cao*), 6g, Fructus Gardeniae Jasminoidis (*Zhi Zi*), 10g, Radix Et Rhizoma Rhei (*Da Huang*), 6g, Radix Et Rhizoma Notopterygii (*Qiang Huo*), 6g, Radix

Ledebouriellae Divaricatae (*Fang Feng*), 6g, Radix Ligustici Wallichii (*Chuan Xiong*), 10g, Radix Angelicae Sinensis (*Dang Gui*), 6g, Folium Bambusae (*Zhu Ye*), 10g

5. Lung yin vacuity

Symptoms: Dry throat often accompanied by an itchy throat and dry nose, red mucous membranes of the pharynx. Other symptoms may include dry cough with no or scant, sticky phlegm, possible hoarse voice, a red tongue with thin, white fur, and a fine, rapid pulse.

Therapeutic principles: Enrich and nourish lung yin

Acupuncture & moxibustion:

Lie Que (Lu 7) *Zhao Hai* (Ki 6)	Together, these points enrich yin and moisten the throat.
Zhong Fu (Lu 1) *Fei Shu* (Bl 13)	A combination of transporting and alarm points; together, they nourish lung yin.
San Yin Jiao (Sp 6)	Nourishes yin to help moisten the throat

Chinese medicinal formula: *Bai He Gu Jin Tang* (Lily Secure Metal Decoction)

Ingredients: Bulbus Lilii (*Bai He*), 10g, uncooked Radix Rehmanniae (*Sheng Di*), 10g, prepared Radix Rehmanniae (*Shu Di*), 12g, Tuber Ophiopogonis Japonici (*Mai Dong*), 10g, Rhizoma Anemarrhenae Asphodeloidis (*Zhi Mu*), 10g, Radix Scrophulariae Ningpoensis (*Xuan Shen*), 10g, Radix Platycodi Grandiflori (*Jie Geng*), 6g, Radix Angelicae Sinensis (*Dang Gui*), 6g, Radix Albus Paeoniae Lactiflorae (*Bai Shao*), 6g, Radix Glycyrrhizae (*Gan Cao*), 6g

6. Kidney yin vacuity

Symptoms: Dry throat often accompanied by a dry root of the tongue. Other symptoms may include tinnitus and deafness, dizziness and vertigo, low back and knee pain and weakness, seminal emission, insomnia, spontaneous perspiration or night sweats, a red tongue with scant fur, and a fine, rapid pulse.

Therapeutic principles: Enrich yin and supplement the kidneys

Acupuncture & moxibustion:

Ren Ying (St 9)	Together, these points nourish yin and moisten the throat. Tap all these points with a plum blossom needle 3-5 times on each point.
Tai Xi (Ki 3)	
Shen Shu (Bl 23)	
San Yin Jiao (Sp 6)	
Zhao Hai (Ki 6)	

Chinese medicinal formula: Modified *Liu Wei Di Huang Wan* (Six Flavors Rehmannia Pills)

Ingredients: Prepared Radix Rehmanniae (*Shu Di*), 12g, Fructus Corni Officinalis (*Shan Zhu Yu*), 10g, Radix Dioscoreae Oppositae (*Shan Yao*), 10g, Sclerotium Poriae Cocos (*Fu Ling*), 6g, Rhizoma Alismatis (*Ze Xie*), 6g, Cortex Radicis Moutan (*Dan Pi*), 6g, Radix Scrophulariae Ningpoensis (*Xuan Shen*), 10g, Tuber Asparagi Cochinensis (*Tian Dong*), 10g

39
Hoarse Voice *(Sheng Yin Si Ya)*

Hoarse voice refers to a relatively low, harsh or husky, often muffled or laboriously forced quality to the sound of the voice which has little or no resonance.

Disease causes, disease mechanisms:

Hoarseness can be grossly divided into two patterns: repletion and vacuity. This two-fold division is encompassed by the saying from the classics, "A solid piece of metal makes no sound, neither does a broken hollow piece." The replete pattern is mainly caused by the invasion of external evils which stagnate in the throat, leading to inhibition of the glottis or inhibition of the flow of lung qi. The vacuity pattern is usually caused by vacuity of the lungs, kidneys, and/or spleen, since, as we know, the voice is the sound of the lungs, is rooted in the kidneys, and is supported by the spleen.

1. Wind cold invasion

The normal voice depends on the free flow of the lung qi and uninhibited switching of the voice gate, (*i.e.*, the glottis). If wind cold invades the exterior, this typically results in non-diffusion of the lung qi. If wind cold evils stagnate in the voice gate, the switching of the glottis will be inhibited. Therefore, hoarse voice may occur.

2. Wind heat invasion

If wind heat evils invade the body, the lungs will be affected, leading to impaired lung depuration. In that case, heat evils will congest in the lungs. The throat pertains to the lungs. If this heat goes upward, steaming and binding in the throat, qi stagnation and blood congestion will result locally, thus giving rise to inhibited switching of the glottis. Hence there is hoarse voice.

3. Yin vacuity of the lungs & kidneys

Yin vacuity may arise from constitutional vacuity, taxation, chronic disease, aging, etc. With lung yin vacuity, there will be impaired lung depuration, leading to inhibited lung qi. With kidney yin vacuity, the throat will be deprived of sufficient nourishment. What is worse, yin vacuity fire will typically flame upward, burning and damaging the throat if vacuous yin fails to check yang. If the lung qi becomes inhibited and there is lack of nourishment and damage to the throat, hoarse voice will occur.

4. Qi vacuity of the lungs & spleen

This vacuity may be the result of taxation from speaking or singing, chronic disease, and dietary irregularity. The voice is the sound of the lungs which is rooted in the kidneys and supported by the spleen. Therefore, if there is qi vacuity of the lungs and spleen, the qi flow will not always be strong enough to dash out through the glottis. Thus the voice may become hoarse.

5. Qi stagnation, blood stasis & phlegm congelation

Qi stagnation, blood stasis, and phlegm congelation may be due to lingering evils which bind in the throat after an acute throat disease or they may arise from taxation due to enduring speaking or singing which may damage the network vessels in the throat. They may also be due to stubborn phlegm which hinders and blocks the free and uninhibited flow of qi and blood. If stagnant qi, static blood, or phlegm congelation block the network vessels in the throat or lead to the formation of nodules there, the voice will be hoarse.

Treatment based on pattern discrimination:

I. Wind cold invasion

Symptoms: Abrupt onset of hoarse voice, possible slightly sore or itchy throat, fever with aversion to cold, headache, body aches, nasal congestion, runny nose with clear mucous, absence of sweating and thirst, cough, thin, white tongue fur, and a floating, tight pulse

Therapeutic principles: Resolve the exterior with acrid, warm ingredients, diffuse the lungs and restore the voice

Acupuncture & moxibustion:

Fu Tu (LI 18)	Frees the flow of qi and blood in the throat
He Gu (LI 4) *Wai Guan* (TB 5)	Together, these points course wind, scatter cold, and disinhibit the throat.
Fei Shu (Bl 13)	Prevents wind cold from entering the lungs and clears heat if there is any

Chinese medicinal formula: *San Ao Tang* (Three [Ingredients] Unbinding Decoction)

Ingredients: Herba Ephedrae (*Ma Huang*), 12g, Semen Pruni Armeniacae (*Xing Ren*), 10g, Radix Glycyrrhizae (*Gan Cao*), 6g

2. Wind heat invasion

Symptoms: A hoarse voice which often starts with discomfort in the throat, dry, painful, itchy throat typically followed by a red, sore, swollen throat. Other symptoms may include cough with yellow phlegm, fever, sweating, headache, slightly red tongue edges with yellow fur, and a floating, rapid pulse.

243

Therapeutic principles: Course wind and clear heat, disinhibit the larynx and restore the voice

Acupuncture & moxibustion:

Lian Quan (CV 23)	Frees the flow of channel qi and clears heat in the throat
Lie Que (Lu 7) *He Gu* (LI 4)	A combination of source and network points; together, they course wind and dissipate the heat to disinhibit the throat. In addition, *Lie Que* connects with the conception vessel which, in turn, connects with the throat.

Chinese medicinal formula: *Sang Ju Yin* (Morus & Chrysanthemum Drink)

Ingredients: Folium Mori Albi (*Sang Ye*), 12g, Flos Chrysanthemi Morifolii (*Ju Hua*), 12g, Semen Pruni Armeniacae (*Xing Ren*), 10g, Fructus Forsythiae Suspensae (*Lian Qiao*), 10g, Herba Menthae Haplocalycis (*Bo He*), 6g, Radix Platycodi Grandiflori (*Jie Geng*), 10g, Rhizoma Phragmitis Communis (*Lu Gen*), 10g, Radix Glycyrrhizae (*Gan Cao*), 6g

3. Yin vacuity of the lungs & kidneys

Symptoms: Chronic hoarse voice. The voice is low and speaking takes effort. Enduring speaking may lead to hoarse voice. The hoarseness becomes worse when there is overwork or enduring speaking. Other symptoms may include slight sore throat or discomfort in the throat which the patient tries to relieve by deliberate coughing, possible itching in the throat, a red throat, dry cough with scant phlegm, dizziness, tinnitus, vacuity vexation, reduced sleep, low back and knee pain and weakness, heat in the palms of the hands and soles of the feet, a red tongue with scant fur, and a fine, rapid pulse.

Therapeutic principles: Enrich and nourish the lungs and kidneys, downbear fire, disinhibit the throat, and restore the voice

Acupuncture and moxibustion:

Lie Que (Lu 7)	Together, these points downbear fire and
Zhao Hai (Ki 6)	disinhibit the throat.
San Yin Jiao (Sp 6)	Together, these points nourish yin to downbear
Tai Xi (Ki 3)	yin vacuity fire.

Additions & subtractions: If there is severe sore, swollen throat, add *Yu Ji* (Lu 10).

Chinese medicinal formula: Modified *Bai He Gu Jin Tang* (Lily Secure Metal Decoction)

Ingredients: Uncooked Radix Rehmanniae (*Sheng Di*), 10g, prepared Radix Rehmanniae (*Shu Di*), 12g, Tuber Ophiopogonis Japonici (*Mai Dong*), 10g, Bulbus Lilii (*Bai He*), 10g, Radix Scrophulariae Ningpoensis (*Xuan Shen*), 10g, Radix Astragali Membranacei (*Huang Qi*), 15g, Radix Dioscoreae Oppositae (*Shan Yao*), 10g, Fructus Terminaliae Chebulae (*He Zi*), 10g

4. Qi vacuity of the lungs & spleen

Symptoms: Chronic hoarseness which is worse in the afternoon and is exacerbated by taxation. There is a low voice and speaking takes effort. Prolonged speaking is impossible. Other symptoms may include shortness of breath, disinclination to speak, fatigue, lack of strength, torpid intake, loose stools, red mucous membranes in the throat, pale red lips and tongue, a fat tongue with white fur, and a vacuous, weak pulse.

Therapeutic principles: Supplement and boost the lungs and spleen, boost the qi and restore the voice

Acupuncture & moxibustion:

Tian Ding (LI 17) *Fu Tu* (LI 18)	Together, these points free the flow of qi in the throat.
Shan Zhong (CV 17)	The meeting point of the qi; regulates and supplements the lung qi
Zu San Li (St 36) *Qi Hai* (CV 6)	Together, these points boost the qi to restore the voice.

Chinese medicinal formula: Modified *Si Jun Zi Tang* (Four Gentlemen Decoction)

Ingredients: Radix Panacis Ginseng (*Ren Shen*), 6g, Rhizoma Atractylodis Macrocephalae (*Bai Zhu*), 10g, Sclerotium Poriae Cocos (*Fu Ling*), 10g, Radix Astragali Membranacei (*Huang Qi*), 15g, Fructus Terminaliae Chebulae (*He Zi*), 10g, Rhizoma Acori Graminei (*Shi Chang Pu*), 10g, mix-fried Radix Glycyrrhizae (*Zhi Gan Cao*), 6g

5. Qi stagnation, blood stasis & phlegm congelation

Symptoms: The hoarseness of the voice is chronic and speaking takes effort. There is discomfort and a sensation as if there was a foreign body in the throat. The patient tends to try to relieve this discomfort and sensation by deliberate coughing. On inspection, the vocal cords are often a dull, stagnant color and there are possible nodules or polyps. Other symptoms may include chest oppression, a dull, stagnant tongue, and choppy pulse.

Therapeutic principles: Move the qi and quicken the blood, transform phlegm and restore the voice

Acupuncture & moxibustion:

Yu Ji (Lu 10)	Quickens the blood

He Gu (LI 4)	Together, these points move the qi, quicken the
San Yin Jiao (Sp 6)	blood, and transform stasis.
Ren Ying (St 9)	Together, these points unblock the network
Tian Ding (LI 17)	vessels to free the flow of qi and blood.

Remarks: Acupuncture is very effective for hoarseness, especially sudden hoarseness. It is possible to actually disperse some small nodules on the vocal cords with acupuncture.

Chinese medicinal formula: *Li Yan Zhu Yu Tang* (Disinhibit the Throat & Dispel Stasis Decoction)

Ingredients: Radix Rubrus Paeoniae Lactiflorae (*Chi Shao*), 10g, Flos Carthami Tinctorii (*Hong Hua*), 10g, Radix Cyathulae (*Chuan Niu Xi*), 10g, Rhizoma Pinelliae Ternatae (*Ban Xia*), 10g, Sclerotium Poriae Cocos (*Fu Ling*), 10g, Pericarpium Citri Reticulatae (*Chen Pi*), 10g, Fructus Terminaliae Chebulae (*He Zi*), 10g, Semen Oroxyli Indici (*Mu Hu Die*), 10g, Rhizoma Acori Graminei (*Shi Chang Pu*), 10g, mix-fried Radix Glycyrrhizae (*Zhi Gan Cao*), 6g

40
Blockage & Obstruction in the Throat
(Hou Zhong Geng Zu)

This refers to a sensation in the throat like a plum-pit obstructing the throat and which cannot be relieved by swallowing or coughing. However, there is no sensation of blockage when eating. On inspection, no abnormality can be found in the region of the throat. In clinical practice, most cases are encountered in women. This condition is also called in Chinese plum-pit qi and in Western medicine neurotic esophageal stenosis or globus hystericus.

Disease causes, disease mechanisms:

All patterns of plum-pit qi are due primarily to liver depression/qi stagnation with upward counterflow of qi. However, based on individual constitutional and lifestyle differences, this basic disease mechanism is compounded by any of several other disease mechanisms.

I. Counterflow of liver qi

Counterflow of liver qi mainly comes from emotional disturbance, such as anger or frustration, which causes liver depression/qi stagnation. If this depressed liver qi counterflows upward along the channel and binds in the throat, there will be a sensation of obstruction in the throat.

2. Phlegm congelation & qi stagnation

The liver is the wood viscus, while the spleen is the earth viscus. If the liver is depressed and becomes replete, it will overwhelm the spleen. The spleen thus becomes vacuous and it loses its command over the movement and transformation of liquids. If water dampness collects, it may accumulate and congeal into phlegm. If liver depression results in upward counterflow of the qi, it may draft this phlegm upward with it where it may become lodged in the throat. Hence there is the sensation as if something were stuck in the throat.

3. Yin vacuity, liver depression

If liver depression due to emotional disturbance has endured for a long time and transformed into heat, this heat may consume yin liquids, eventually resulting in yin vacuity. Because "The blood and essence share a common source" and "The liver and kidneys share a common source," if there is yin vacuity, first, there is typically also blood vacuity. Thus the liver is insufficiently nourished and softened, making liver depression even worse. Secondly, yin vacuity below typically gives rise to vacuity fire above. Because fire's nature is to flame upward, this upwardly flaming fire combines with and aggravates the upwardly counterflowing qi due to stagnation. If this upwardly counterflowing qi and vacuity fire bind in the throat, they may cause obstruction locally and hence a feeling of something stuck in the throat.

4. Blood stasis obstructing the network vessels

Because "The qi moves the blood. If the blood moves, the qi moves. If the qi stops, the blood stops," long-term liver depression and qi stagnation often give rise to blood stasis. It is also said, "Enduring disease enters the network vessels." Therefore, if emotional disturbance gives rise to prolonged and enduring liver depression with qi counterflow binding in the region of the throat, over time, this may lead to blood stasis obstructing the network vessels in the throat. Thus there may occur a sensation of obstruction in the throat.

Treatment based on pattern discrimination:

I. Counterflow of liver qi

Symptoms: There is a sensation as if there were a plum-pit stuck in the back of the throat which cannot be relieved by swallowing down or coughing up and which is exacerbated by emotional disturbance. In some cases, this sensation may come and go. There is no sensation of obstruction when eating. Other symptoms may include dizziness, vexation, irascibility, distending fullness in the chest and lateral costal regions, belching, a normal tongue with thin fur, and a wiry pulse.

Therapeutic principles: Course the liver and rectify the qi

Acupuncture & moxibustion:

Tian Tu (CV 22)	Frees the flow of qi in the throat
Qi Men (Liv 14) *Tai Chong* (Liv 3)	Together, these points course the liver and rectify the qi.
Li Gou (Liv 5)	Helps *Qi Men* and *Tai Chong*

Additions & subtractions: If there is distending fullness in the lateral costal regions, add *Zhang Men* (Liv 13). If there is menstrual irregularity, add *San Yin Jiao* (Sp 6).

Chinese medicinal formula: Modified *Shu Li Tang* (Course & Disinhibit Decoction)

Ingredients: Radix Bupleuri (*Chai Hu*), 6g, Fructus Citri Aurantii (*Zhi Ke*), 10g, Flos Pruni Mume (*Lu O Mei*), 10g, Flos Rosae Rugosae (*Mei Gui Hua*), 5g, Fructus Akebiae (*Ba Yue Zha*), 10g, Caulis Perillae Frutescentis (*Su Geng*), 10g, Radix Clematidis Chinensis (*Wei Ling*

Xian), 15g, Radix Scrophulariae Ningpoensis (*Xuan Shen*), 12g, Radix Glycyrrhizae (*Gan Cao*), 3g

Additions & subtractions: If liver depression transforms into heat, add Cortex Radicis Moutan (*Dan Pi*), 10g, Fructus Gardeniae Jasminoidis (*Zhi Zi*), 10g, and Spica Prunellae Vulgaris (*Xia Ku Cao*), 15g. If there is insomnia, heart palpitations, or vexation and agitation, add Cortex Albizziae Julibrissinis (*He Huan Pi*), 20g, Radix Polygalae Tenuifoliae (*Yuan Zhi*), 10g, and Fructus Schisandrae Chinensis (*Wu Wei Zi*), 10g. If there is dizziness and vertigo due to liver hyperactivity, add Ramulus Uncariae Cum Uncis (*Gou Teng*), 10g, and Fructus Tribuli Terrestris (*Bai Ji Li*), 10g. If there is thick phlegm in the back of the throat which cannot be expectorated, add Fructus Arctii Lappae (*Niu Bang Zi*), 10g, and Bulbus Fritillariae Thunbergii (*Zhe Bei Mu*), 10g. And if there is marked spleen vacuity with damp accumulation and torpid intake, delete Radix Glycyrrhizae (*Gan Cao*) and add scorched Rhizoma Atractylodis Macrocephalae (*Bai Zhu*), 10g, Radix Dioscoreae Oppositae (*Shan Yao*), 10g, and Massa Medica Fermentata (*Shen Qu*), 15g.

2. Phlegm congelation & qi stagnation

Symptoms: The sensation of obstruction comes and goes. Other symptoms may include profuse, sticky phlegm which is difficult to expectorate, fullness in the stomach and abdomen, possible nausea and vomiting, chest oppression, torpid intake, slimy tongue fur, and a soggy, slippery or slippery, wiry pulse.

Therapeutic principles: Move the qi and transform phlegm. However, if phlegm is combined with heat as manifest by a red throat, a bitter taste in the mouth, cough with sticky, yellow phlegm, slimy, yellow tongue fur, and a slippery, rapid pulse, then transform phlegm and clear heat.

Acupuncture & moxibustion:

Tian Tu (CV 22)　　　　Downbears the qi and disinhibits the throat

He Gu (LI 4)   Moves the qi to help transform phlegm

Tai Chong (Liv 3)   Courses the liver and rectifies the qi

Feng Long (St 40)   Together, these points transform phlegm.
Zhong Wan (CV 12)

Additions & subtractions: Add *Nei Guan* (Per 6) if there is fullness and oppression in the chest and diaphragm.

Chinese medicinal formulas:

For phlegm congelation & qi stagnation: Modified *Ban Xia Hou Po Tang* (Pinellia & Magnolia Decoction)

Ingredients: Rhizoma Pinelliae Ternatae (*Ban Xia*), 10g, Cortex Magnoliae Officinalis (*Hou Po*), 10g, Sclerotium Poriae Cocos (*Fu Ling*), 10g, Caulis Perillae Frutescentis (*Su Geng*), 10g, Radix Bupleuri (*Chai Hu*), 6g, Fructus Citri Aurantii (*Zhi Ke*), 10g, Pericarpium Citri Reticulatae (*Chen Pi*), 6g, Radix Clematidis Chinensis (*Wei Ling Xian*), 12g, mix-fried Radix Glycyrrhizae (*Zhi Gan Cao*), 6g

For phlegm heat: Modified *Wen Dan Tang* (Warm the Gallbladder Decoction)

Ingredients: Rhizoma Pinelliae Ternatae (*Ban Xia*), 10g, Pericarpium Citri Reticulatae (*Chen Pi*), 6g, Sclerotium Poriae Cocos (*Fu Ling*), 10g, Fructus Immaturus Citri Aurantii (*Zhi Shi*), 10g, Caulis Bambusae In Taeniis (*Zhu Ru*), 10g, Fructus Trichosanthis Kirlowii (*Tian Hua Fen*), 10g, Bulbus Fritillariae Thunbergii (*Zhe Bei Mu*), 10g, Tuber Curcumae (*Yu Jin*), 10g, Spica Prunellae Vulgaris (*Xia Ku Cao*), 15g, Radix Scutellariae Baicalensis (*Huang Qin*), 12g, Rhizoma Belamcandae (*She Gan*), 10g

Additions & subtractions: If there is lack of appetite, chest and stomach fullness and oppression, and a slimy tongue coating, add Massa Medica

Fermentata (*Shen Qu*), 20g, Endothelium Corneum Gigeriae Galli (*Ji Nei Jin*), 10g, and stir-fried Fructus Germinatus Hordei Vulgaris (*Mai Ya*), 10g. If there is an upper respiratory tract infection, add Flos Lonicerae Japonicae (*Yin Hua*), 15g, Radix Isatidis Seu Baphicacanthi (*Ban Lan Gen*), 15g, and Herba Cum Radice Taraxaci Mongolici (*Pu Gong Ying*), 25g.

3. Yin vacuity, liver depression

Symptoms: A sensation of something obstructing the throat which can neither be coughed up nor swallowed down, a dry mouth and throat, heat in the palms of the hands and soles of the feet, lingering pain in the lateral costal region, a red tongue with scant fur, and a wiry, fine, rapid pulse

Therapeutic principles: Supplement the kidneys and enrich yin, harmonize the liver and downbear counterflow

Acupuncture & moxibustion:

Tian Tu (CV 2)	Frees the flow of qi in the throat
Lie Que (Lu 7) *Zhao Hai* (Ki 6)	Together, these points enrich yin and downbear fire, disinhibit and moisten the throat.
Tai Xi (Ki 3) *San Yin Jiao* (Sp 6)	Together, these points supplement the kidneys and enrich yin.
Tai Chong (Liv 3) *Qu Quan* (Liv 8)	Together, these points harmonize the liver and rectify the qi.

Chinese medicinal formula: Modified *Yi Guan Jian* (One Link Decoction)

Ingredients: Fructus Meliae Toosendan (*Chuan Lian Zi*), 10g, Radix Glehniae Littoralis (*Bei Sha Shen*), 12g, Tuber Ophiopogonis Japonici

(*Mai Dong*), 12g, uncooked Radix Rehmanniae (*Sheng Di*), 12g, Fructus Lycii Chinensis (*Gou Qi Zi*), 10g, Radix Angelicae Sinensis (*Dang Gui*), 10g, Radix Scrophulariae Ningpoensis (*Xuan Shen*), 10g, Tuber Curcumae (*Yu Jin*), 10g, Radix Platycodi Grandiflori (*Jie Geng*), 6g, Radix Albus Paeoniae Lactiflorae (*Bai Shao*), 10g

Additions & subtractions: If there is insomnia or the spirit is disquieted, add Semen Biotae Orientalis (*Bai Zi Ren*), 10g, and stir-fried Semen Zizyphi Spinosae (*Suan Zao Ren*), 20g.

4. Blood stasis obstructing the network vessels

Symptoms: A feeling of something obstructing the throat which can neither be coughed up nor swallowed down, difficulty eating but no trouble drinking water, piercing pain in the chest and lateral costal regions which, if serious, radiates to the upper back, a long disease course, a dark tongue with possible static spots or macules, and a wiry, fine, choppy pulse

Therapeutic principles: Transform stasis and open the network vessels, move the qi and disinhibit the throat

Acupuncture & moxibustion:

Tian Tu (CV 22)	Frees the flow of qi in the throat
Ge Shu (Bl 17) *Xue Hai* (Sp 10)	Together, these points quicken the blood and transform stasis.
He Gu (LI 4) *Tai Chong* (Liv 3)	Together, these points course the liver and rectify the qi.

In addition, prick to bleed any visibly and abnormally engorged and purplish venules found anywhere on the surface of the body.

Chinese medicinal formula: Modified *Xue Fu Zhu Yu Tang* (Blood Mansion Dispel Stasis Decoction)

Ingredients: Semen Pruni Persicae (*Tao Ren*), 10g, Flos Carthami Tinctorii (*Hong Hua*), 10g, Radix Angelicae Sinensis (*Dang Gui*), 10g, Radix Ligustici Wallichii (*Chuan Xiong*), 10g, Radix Rubrus Paeoniae Lactiflorae (*Chi Shao*), 10g, Radix Bupleuri (*Chai Hu*), 10g, Fructus Immaturus Citri Aurantii (*Zhi Shi*), 6g, Radix Platycodi Grandiflori (*Jie Geng*), 6g, Radix Cyathulae (*Chuan Niu Xi*), 10g, Tuber Curcumae (*Yu Jin*), 10g, Spica Prunellae Vulgaris (*Xia Ku Cao*), 10g, Radix Salviae Miltiorrhizae (*Dan Shen*), 10g

Additions & subtractions: If there is a dry, sore throat, add Radix Scrophulariae Ningpoensis (*Xuan Shen*), 15g, Radix Trichosanthis Kirlowii (*Tian Hua Fen*), 15g, and mix-fried Folium Eriobotryae Japonicae (*Pi Pa Ye*), 10g. If there is an itchy throat, add Rhizoma Belamcandae (*She Gan*), 10g, and Herba Menthae Haplocalycis (*Bo He*), 10g. If there is a feeling as if something is stuck in the throat, add Caulis Perillae Frutescentis (*Su Geng*), 10g, and Rhizoma Pinelliae Ternatae (*Ban Xia*), 10g.

Bibliography

Chinese language:

Lin Chuang Bian Zheng Shi Zhi Xue (A Study of the Clinical Basing of Treatment on Pattern Discrimination) by Liu Bin, Science, Technology & Literature Press, Beijing, 1992

Shi Yong Zhong Yi Zhen Duan Xue (A Study of Practical Chinese Medicine Diagnosis) by Liu Tie-Tiao, Shanghai Science & Technology Press, Shanghai, 1988

Zhong Yi Bi Bing Da Quan (A Compendium of Chinese Medicine Nose Diseases) by Lu Xiao-zuo and Jiang Xian-yang, Tianjin Science & Technology Press, Tianjin, 1995

Zhong Yi Bing Yin Bing Ji Xue (A Study of Chinese Medicine Disease Causes & Disease Mechanisms) by Song Lu-bing, People's Health & Hygiene Press, Beijing, 1987

Zhong Yi Da Ci Dian, Nei Ke Fen Ce (Encyclopedia of Chinese Medicine, Volume on Internal Medicine), People's Health & Hygiene Press, Beijing, 1987

Zhong Yi Da Ci Dian, Wu Guan Ke Fen Ce (Encyclopedia of Chinese Medicine: Volume on the Five Sense Organs) People's Health & Hygiene Press, Beijing, 1988

Zhong Yi Er Bi Hou Ke Xue (A Study of Chinese Medicine Otonasaolaryngology) by Tan Jing-shu, Hunan Science & Technology Press, Changsha, 1989

Zhong Yi Er Bi Yan Hou Kou Qiang Xue (A Study of Chinese Medicine E.N.T. and Stomatology) by Wang De-jian, People's Health a Hygiene Press, Beijing, 1994

Zhong Yi Nei Ke Xue (A Study of Chinese Medicine Internal Medicine) by Zhang Bo-Yu, People's Health & Hygiene Press, Beijing, 1988

Zhong Yi Nei Ke Zheng Zhuang Bian Zhi Shou Ce (A Handbook of Chinese Medicine Internal Medicine Symptoms Discrimination & Treatment) by Fang Wen-xian, Liu Qing & Chu Xiu-jun, China Standard Press, Beijing, 1989

Zhong Yi Wu Guan Ke Xue (A Study of the Chinese Medicine Specialty in the Five Sense Organs) by the Guang Zhou College of Chinese Medicine, People's Health & Hygiene Press, Beijing, 1991

Zhong Yi Yan Ke Xue (A Study of Chinese Medicine Ophthalmology) by the Guangzhou College of Chinese Medicine, Shanghai Science & Technology Press, Shanghai, 1981

Zhang Yi Yan Ke Xue (A Study of Chinese Medicine Ophthalmology) by Liao Pin-zheng, Shanghai Science and Technology Press, Shanghai, 1986

Zhong Yi Yan Ke Xue (A Study of Chinese Medicine Ophthalmology) by the Chengdu college of Chinese Medicine, People's Health & Hygiene Press, Beijing, 1985

Zhong Yi Zheng Hou Zhen Duan Zhi Liao Xue (A Study of Chinese Medicine Patterns, Diagnosis & Treatment) by Cheng Shao-en & Xia Hong-sheng, Beijing Science & Technology Press, Beijing, 1993

Zhong Yi Zheng Zhuang Jian Bie Zhen Duan Xue (A Study of Chinese Medicine Symptoms & Differential Diagnosis) by Zhao Jin-ze, People's Health & Hygiene Press, Beijing, 1984

Zhong Yi Zhi Liao Xue (A Study of Chinese Medicine Treatments) by Sun Guo-jie & Tu Jin-wen, China Medicine & Medicinals Science & Technology Press, Beijing, 1990

English language:

Chinese Acupuncture & Moxibustion edited by Cheng Xin-nong, Foreign Languages Press, Beijing, 1987

Chinese Herbal Medicine: Formulas & Strategies by Dan Bensky & Randall Barolet, Eastland Press, Seattle, 1990

Chinese Herbal Medicine: Materia Medica by Dan Bensky & Andrew Gamble, Eastland Press, Seattle, 1993

Fundamentals of Chinese Acupuncture by Andrew Ellis, Nigel Wiseman & Ken Boss, Paradigm Publications, Brookline, MA, 1988

Fundamentals of Chinese Medicine translated & amended by Nigel Wiseman & Andrew Ellis, Paradigm Publications, Brookline, MA, 1985

Glossary of Chinese Medical Terms and Acupuncture Points by Nigel Wiseman, Paradigm Publications, Brookline, Ma, 1990

Pao Zhi: An Introduction to the Use of Processed Chinese Medicinals by Philippe Sionneau, Blue Poppy Press, Boulder, CO, 1995

Seventy Essential TCM Formulas for Beginners by Bob Flaws, Blue Poppy Press, Boulder, CO, 1994

Statements of Fact in TCM by Bob Flaws, Blue Poppy Press, Boulder, CO, 1994

Other books by Philippe Sionneau

L'Acupuncture Pratiquée en Chine, Vol. 1: Les Points Traditionels, Guy Tredaniel Editeur, Paris, 1994

L'Acupuncture Pratiquée en Chine, Vol. 2: Les Traitments Efficaces, Guy Tredaniel Editeur, Paris, 1994

Pao Zhi: An Introduction to the Use of Processed Chinese Medicinals, translated by Bob Flaws, Blue Poppy Press, Boulder, CO, 1994

Troubles Psychologiques et Psychiatriques en Médecine Chinoise, Editions Rouergue, forthcoming in 1996

Utilization Clinique de la Pharmocopée Chinoise, Vol. 1: Les Substances Médicinales Preparée, So Dai Editions, Paris, 1994

Utilization Clinique de la Pharmacopée Chinoise, Vol. 2: Traitment Efficaces: Selection des Substances Médicinales-cles, Editions Rouergue, forthcoming in 1996

Formula Index

A, B

An Gong Niu Huang Wan 108
Ba Zhen Tang 88, 131, 194
Bai He Gu Jin Tang 163, 231, 238, 245
Ban Xia Hou Po Tang 253
Ban Xia Tian Ma Bai Zhu Tang 15
Bu Shen Ci Shi Wan 83
Bu Xin Dan 17
Bu Zhong Yi Qi Tang 18, 35, 101, 126, 164, 180

C

Cang Er Zi San 177, 180, 184, 189
Chai Hu Shen Zhu Tang 4, 102
Chu Feng Yi Sun Tang 36
Chu Shi Tang 10, 168, 205
Chuan Xiong Cha Tiao San 44
Cong Rong Wan 124

D

Da Huang Dang Gui San 76
Dan Zhi Xiao Yao San 94
Dao Chi San 78
Di Tan Tang 109
Ding Zhi Wan 83

E, F, G

Er Long Zuo Ci Wan 123
Fu Zi Li Zhong Tang 199
Gou Qi Zi Jiu 51
Gui Pi Tang 31, 155

H

Hua Jian Er Chen Wan 40
Huang Lian E Jiao Tang 125
Huang Lian Wen Dan Tang 127
Huang Qin Hua Shi Tang 179, 198

Huo Xiang Zheng Qi San 172

J

Jia Wei Si Ling San 178
Jia Wei Xiao Yao San 4
Ju Hua Tong Shen San 64
Ju Jing Wan 52

L, M

Li Yan Zhu Yu Tang 247
Li Zhong Tang 199, 214
Lian Qiao Yin Zi 58
Liang Ge San 10
Ling Yang Jiao San 49
Liu Wei Di Huang Wan 87, 198, 239
Liu Wei Tang 229
Long Dan Xie Gan Tang 29, 69, 110, 121, 130, 136, 137, 142, 154, 190, 196
Ma Huang Tang 151
Ming Mu Xi Xin Tang 57

P, Q

Pu Ji Xiao Du Yin 135
Qi Ju Di Huang Wan 50, 95, 100
Qiang Huo Sheng Feng Tang 64
Qing Jin San 204
Qing Tan Yin 74
Qing Wei San 162, 174, 237
Qing Wei Tang 41, 232
Qing Yan Li Ge Tang 218, 223
Qing Ying Tang 107, 204
Qing Zao Jiu Fei Tang 23, 161, 167, 236
Qu Feng San 7, 65
Qu Feng San Re Yin Zi 65
Qu Yu Si Wu Tang 37

R, S

Ren Shen Qiang Huo Tang 9

261

General Index

facial complexion, white, lusterless 122
facial swelling 30
far-sightedness 85, 86, 90
fatigue 17, 22, 30, 31, 72, 124, 126, 131, 134, 143, 179, 191, 198, 221, 245
fauces, redness and swelling of the isthmus of the 222
fever 2, 27, 44, 63, 69, 74, 87, 107, 111, 119, 125, 130, 134, 135, 140-142, 151, 160, 161, 163, 166, 172, 173, 176, 177, 182, 183, 188, 189, 202-204, 208, 216, 217, 221, 222, 228-231, 234, 235, 243
fever, alternating chills and 217
fever, high 27, 107, 142, 173, 202, 203, 217, 222
fever, high, persistent 217
fever, low-grade 231
fever, tidal 69, 87, 111, 125, 163
fever, tidal, with red cheeks 111
food intake, diminished 15, 18, 31, 75, 92, 95, 101, 108, 113, 124, 126, 168, 191, 213
food, no thought of 198

H

head, cloudedness and distention in the 191
head, distention in the 76, 153, 184, 191
headache 2, 28, 35, 43, 45, 49, 52, 63, 68, 78, 87, 109, 113, 119, 120, 127, 134, 135, 140, 141, 146, 151, 160, 161, 166, 173, 176-178, 183, 189, 190, 192, 196, 197, 202, 204, 209, 211, 216, 221, 228, 229, 235, 243
headache, severe 192
heart palpitations 4, 17, 31, 82, 88, 95, 99, 102, 112, 125, 147, 155, 193, 252
heart, racing of the 31, 88
heat, aversion to 68
heat in the palms of the hands and soles of the feet 218, 223, 244, 254
heavy-headedness 92, 108, 178, 209

hypopsia 91

I, J

impotence 19, 83, 101, 124
inability to see objects clearly after sunset 99, 101
insomnia 4, 17, 22, 31, 45, 52, 79, 88, 102, 121, 123, 125, 219, 224, 239, 252, 255
irascibility 45, 110, 146, 153, 205, 251
itching in the canthi 6
itchy eyes 5, 8, 10, 23, 29, 35, 99
itchy throat 163, 227-232, 238, 243, 256
joints, aching in the 44

L

lateral costal pain 3, 16, 68, 75, 93, 109, 120, 254
lateral costal pain and distention 68, 112
limbs, chilled 19, 89, 101, 124, 143, 213
limbs, convulsive spasm of the 203
limbs, counterflow frigidity of the 156
lips and nails, pale 4, 50
lips, thirst with dry 161
low back ache 22, 198
low back and knee pain and weakness 18, 30, 52, 69, 73, 80, 83, 86, 87, 94, 100, 101, 110, 121, 124, 125, 147, 155, 219, 224, 239, 244
low back pain and lack of strength 132
lower limbs, fear of cold in the 58

M

maculopapular eruptions 107
malaise, general 151, 160, 161
memory, impaired 31
middle ear, pain in the 134
mouth and throat, dry 23, 41, 48, 58, 72, 78, 86, 121, 123, 160, 162, 167, 196, 254

otopyorrhea 139, 140

perspiration, spontaneous 4, 19, 102, 164, 168, 239

phlegm, profuse 15, 92, 127, 186, 189, 209

photophobia 7, 27, 43, 45, 55-59, 63, 65, 66, 99

plum-pit qi 249

premature ejaculation 19, 80, 101

pupils, dilatation of the 71-76

pyretophobia 55-59

R

ringing which sounds like a tide 126

runny nose 56, 140, 172, 173, 175, 176, 178, 179, 182-184, 186-192, 196, 208-211, 229, 243

runny nose precipitated by cold 179

runny nose with clear mucous 172, 182, 229, 243

runny nose with profuse, yellow, turbid discharge 178

runny nose with sticky, yellow mucous 184

runny nose with turbid mucous 173

runny nose with white, sticky nasal mucous 191

runny nose with yellow mucous 183

runny nose with yellow-green nasal mucous 196

S

scabs on the nasal mucous membranes 164

seeing large things as small 92

skin, drained white 30

sleep, desire for 197, 198

sleep, reduced 72, 100, 244

sleeping, profuse 15

smell, decreased sense of 161, 178, 184-186, 187-189, 191, 196, 209

sneezing 166, 168, 176, 182, 229

sneezing, frequent 16 6, 168, 176

spasm of the limbs, convulsive 203

speak, disinclination to 154, 179, 191, 231, 245

speech, delirious 107

spirit, clouded, and delirium 107, 203

spirit, lassitude of the 82, 88, 95, 101, 102, 111, 147, 154, 164, 197, 210, 218, 223

stomach, clamoring 162, 236

stomach, fullness and oppression in the chest and 126

stomach, fullness in the 113, 168, 172, 178, 179, 252

stomach, painful, burning heat in the 236

stools, dry 9, 135, 141, 160, 162, 196, 217, 232, 236

strength, lack of 18, 30, 31, 34, 72, 101, 102, 124, 126, 131, 132, 147, 154, 164, 168, 179, 189, 193, 197, 198, 211, 245

submaxillary nodes 222

superciliary arch, pain or aching in the 2

swallowing, difficulty 222

sweating 149, 151, 156, 160, 176, 177, 183, 216, 227, 228, 231, 243

sweating, absence of 176, 243

sweating, profuse 156

sweats, night 18, 69, 80, 86, 87, 112, 123, 125, 155, 156, 163, 239

T

taste in the mouth, bitter 3, 9, 16, 28, 68, 92, 93, 108-110, 113, 120, 135, 136, 141, 146, 153, 189, 237, 252

tearing 3, 7, 8, 47-52, 57, 63, 66-68

tearing in the wind 47, 48, 50, 57

tearing, persistent cold 52

tears, hot 9, 10, 27

teeth, loosening of the 86

thin, clear, odorless pus 142

thirst, vexatious, with a desire to drink 152

STICKING TO THE POINT: A Rational Methodology for the Step by Step Formulation & Administration of an Acupuncture Treatment by Bob Flaws ISBN 0-936185-17-1 $16.95

ENDOMETRIOSIS, INFERTILITY AND TRADITIONAL CHINESE MEDICINE: A Laywoman's Guide by Bob Flaws ISBN 0-936185-14-7 $9.95

THE BREAST CONNECTION: A Laywoman's Guide to the Treatment of Breast Disease by Chinese Medicine by Honora Lee Wolfe ISBN 0-936185-61-9, $9.95

NINE OUNCES: A Nine Part Program For The Prevention of AIDS in HIV Positive Persons by Bob Flaws ISBN 0-936185-12-0 $9.95

THE TREATMENT OF CANCER BY INTEGRATED CHINESE-WESTERN MEDICINE by Zhang Dai-zhao, trans. by Zhang Ting-liang & Bob Flaws, ISBN 0-936185-11-2, $18.95

A HANDBOOK OF TRADITIONAL CHINESE DERMATOLOGY by Liang Jian-hui, trans. by Zhang Ting-liang & Bob Flaws, ISBN 0-936185-07-4 $15.95

A HANDBOOK OF TRADITIONAL CHINESE GYNECOLOGY by Zhejiang College of TCM, trans. by Zhang Ting-liang, ISBN 0-936185-06-6 (4nd edit.) $22.95

PRINCE WEN HUI'S COOK: Chinese Dietary Therapy by Bob Flaws & Honora Lee Wolfe, ISBN 0-

912111-05-4, $12.95 (Published by Paradigm Press, Brookline, MA)

THE DAO OF INCREASING LONGEVITY AND CONSERVING ONE'S LIFE by Anna Lin & Bob Flaws, ISBN 0-936185-24-4 $16.95

FIRE IN THE VALLEY: The TCM Diagnosis and Treatment of Vaginal Diseases by Bob Flaws ISBN 0-936185-25-2 $16.95

HIGHLIGHTS OF ANCIENT ACUPUNCTURE PRESCRIPTIONS trans. by Honora Lee Wolfe & Rose Crescenz ISBN 0-936185-23-6, $14.95

ARISAL OF THE CLEAR: A Simple Guide to Healthy Eating According to Traditional Chinese Medicine by Bob Flaws, ISBN #-936185-27-9 $8.95

PEDIATRIC BRONCHITIS: Its Cause, Diagnosis & Treatment According to Traditional Chinese Medicine trans. by Gao Yu-li and Bob Flaws, ISBN 0-936185-26-0 $15.95

AIDS & ITS TREATMENT ACCORDING TO TRADITIONAL CHINESE MEDICINE by Huang Bing-shan, trans. by Fu-Di & Bob Flaws, ISBN 0-936185-28-7 $24.95

ACUTE ABDOMINAL SYNDROMES: Their Diagnosis & Treatment by Combined Chinese-Western Medicine by Alon Marcus, ISBN 0-936185-31-7 $16.95

MY SISTER, THE MOON: The Diagnosis & Treatment of Menstrual Diseases by Traditional Chinese Medicine by Bob Flaws, ISBN 0-936185-34-1, $24.95

FU QING-ZHU'S GYNE-COLOGY trans. by Yang Shou-zhong and Liu Da-wei, ISBN 0-936185-35-X, $22.95

FLESHING OUT THE BONES: The Importance of Case Histories in Chinese Medicine trans. by Charles Chace. ISBN 0-936185-30-9, $18.95

CLASSICAL MOXIBUSTION SKILLS in Contemporary Clinical Practice by Sung Baek, ISBN 0-936185-16-3 $12.95

THE MEDICAL I CHING: Oracle of the Healer Within by Miki Shima, OMD, ISBN 0-936185-38-4, $19.95

MASTER TONG'S ACUPUNC-TURE: An Ancient Lineage for Modern Practice, trans. and commentary by Miriam Lee, OMD, ISBN 0-936185-37-6, $19.95

A HANDBOOK OF TCM UROL-OGY & MALE SEXUAL DYSFUNCTION by Anna Lin, OMD, ISBN 0-936185-36-8, $16.95

MASTER HUA'S CLASSIC OF THE CENTRAL VISCERA by Hua Tuo, ISBN 0-936185-43-0, $21.95

THE HEART & ESSENCE OF DAN-XI'S METHODS OF TREATMENT by Xu Dan-xi, trans. by Yang Shou-zhong, ISBN 0-926185-49-X, $21.95

STATEMENTS OF FACT IN TRADITIONAL CHINESE MEDICINE by Bob Flaws, ISBN 0-936185-52-X, $12.95

IMPERIAL SECRETS OF HEALTH & LONGEVITY by Bob Flaws, ISBN 0-936185-51-1, $9.95

THE SYSTEMATIC CLASSIC OF ACUPUNCTURE & MOXIBUS-TION (*Jia Yi Jing*) by Huang-fu Mi, trans. by Yang Shou-zhong and Charles Chace, ISBN 0-936185-29-5, $79.95

CHINESE MEDICINAL WINES & ELIXIRS by Bob Flaws, ISBN 0-936185-58-9, $18.95

THE DIVINELY RESPONDING CLASSIC: A Translation of the *Shen Ying Jing* from *Zhen Jiu Da Cheng*, trans. by Yang Shou-zhong & Liu Feng-ting ISBN 0-936185-55-4, $15.95

PAO ZHI: An Introduction to Processing Chinese Medicinals to Enhance Their Therapeutic Effect, by Philippe Sionneau, ISBN 0-936185-62-1, $34.95

THE BOOK OF JOOK: Chinese Medicinal Porridges, An Alternative to the Typical Western Breakfast, by Bob Flaws, ISBN0-936185-60-0, $16.95

SHAOLIN SECRET FORMULAS for the Treatment of External Injuries, by De Chan, ISBN 0-936185-08-2, $18.95

AGING & BLOOD STASIS: A New Approach to TCM Geriatrics, by Yan De-xin, ISBN 0-936185-63-5, $21.95

CHINESE MEDICAL PALM-ISTRY: Your Health in Your Hand, by Zong Xiao-fan & Gary Liscum, ISBN 0-936185-64-3, $15.95

THE SECRET OF CHINESE PULSE DIAGNOSIS by Bob Flaws, ISBN 0-936185-67-8, $17.95

LOW BACK PAIN: Care & Prevention with Traditional Chinese Medicine by Douglas Frank, ISBN 0-936185-66-X, $9.95

A COMPENDIUM OF TCM PATTERNS & TREATMENTS by Bob Flaws & Daniel Finney, ISBN 0-936185-70-8, $29.95

ACUPUNCTURE AND MOXIBUSTION FORMULAS & TREATMENTS by Cheng Dan-an, trans. By Wu Ming, ISBN 0-936185-68-6, $22.95

THE TREATMENT OF DISEASE IN TCM, Vol I: Diseases of the Head & Face Including Mental/Emotional Disorders by Philippe Sionneau & Lü Gang, ISBN 0-936185-69-4, $21.95

KEEPING YOUR CHILD HEALTHY WITH CHINESE MEDICINE: A Parent's Guide to the Care and Prevention of Common Childhood Diseases, by Bob Flaws, ISBN 0-936185-71-6, $15.95